Pharmaceutical Inorganic Chemistry (BP104T)

(As per Pharmacy Council of India Syllabus)

Bachelor of Pharmacy

(1st Semester)

I0479407

Author

Priyanka Panth
Associate Professor
M.S. College of Pharmacy

Preface

Pharmaceutical Inorganic Chemistry is a dynamic and rapidly evolving field that plays a critical role in the development of new drugs and therapies. The study of inorganic compounds and their applications in the pharmaceutical industry is essential for understanding the complex processes involved in the synthesis and characterization of these compounds. This syllabus provides a comprehensive overview of the fundamental principles of inorganic chemistry and its applications in the pharmaceutical industry.

The syllabus is divided into five units, each covering a different aspect of the field.

Unit I cover impurities in pharmaceutical substances, including their sources, types, and the principle involved in limit tests.

Unit II focuses on acids, bases, and buffers, as well as major extra and intracellular electrolytes and dental products.

Unit III examines gastrointestinal agents, including acidifiers, antacids, cathartics, and antimicrobials.

Unit IV covers miscellaneous compounds, including expectorants, emetics, haematinics, poison and antidotes, and astringents.

Unit V discusses radiopharmaceuticals, including radioactivity, radioisotopes, and their pharmaceutical applications.

This syllabus is designed for students with a background in general and inorganic chemistry who are interested in pursuing careers in the pharmaceutical industry or who simply wish to expand their knowledge in the field. The course emphasizes the development of critical thinking skills and the application of knowledge to real-world problems.

We hope that this syllabus will provide students with a solid foundation in the principles of inorganic chemistry and its applications in the pharmaceutical industry and inspire them to continue their studies in this exciting and challenging field.

Acknowledgement

The successful completion of this book would not have been possible without the support and guidance of several individuals. First and foremost, I would like to express my deep gratitude to **Dr Mohammad Hashim Mansoori, Principal** of **M.S. College of Pharmacy, Devghar, Tal. Wada, Dist. Palghar (MH)** who provided invaluable support and guidance throughout the writing process. Their encouragement, insight, and unwavering faith in my abilities were instrumental in bringing this book to fruition.

I would also like to extend my heartfelt thanks to **M.S. College of Pharmacy, Devghar, Tal. Wada, Dist. Palghar (MH)**, for providing me with the opportunity to develop my expertise in the field of pharmaceutical inorganic chemistry and for supporting my research. I am deeply grateful for the many colleagues and classmates who have contributed to my education and provided me with invaluable feedback on this book.

I would like to express my gratitude to my Husband **Dr Kapil Raghav** who has provided me with the love, support, and encouragement I needed to complete this project. Their unwavering support and encouragement have been a source of inspiration and strength throughout the writing process.

I would also like to specifically acknowledge the contributions of the following colleagues who have made significant contributions to this book: Ashwin Somkuwar, Sameer Khan, Ainulsha Feeque,

Priyanka Bushara, TarannumSathi, Rupali Bhoir, Abhishek Shelar, Varsha Ghodake, Nushrat Khan, Mahreen Falke.

These individuals have shared their knowledge, expertise, and guidance in the field of pharmaceutical inorganic chemistry, and endeavour contributions have greatly enriched the content of this book. I am grateful for their time, dedication, and commitment to this project.

This book is dedicated to all of the individuals who have contributed to my education and growth as a researcher and writer. Thank you for your unwavering support and guidance.

Priyanka Panth
Associate Professor
MS College of Pharmacy,
Devghar, Dist. Palghar, (MH)

(BP104T) PHARMACEUTICAL INORGANIC CHEMISTRY
(Theory)

45 Hours

Course Content:

UNIT-I
10 Hours

•**Impurities in pharmaceutical substances:** History of Pharmacopoeia, Sources and types of impurities, principle involved in the limit test for Chloride, Sulphate, Iron, Arsenic, Lead and Heavy metals, modified limit test for Chloride and Sulphate

General methods of preparation, assay for the compounds superscripted with asterisk (*), properties and medicinal uses of inorganic compounds belonging to the following classes.

UNIT-II
10 Hours

• **Acids, Bases and Buffers:** Buffer equations and buffer capacity in general, buffers in pharmaceutical systems, preparation, stability, buffered isotonic solutions, measurements of tonicity, calculations and methods of adjusting isotonicity.

• **Major extra and intracellular electrolytes:** Functions of major physiological ions, Electrolytes used in the replacement therapy: Sodium chloride*, Potassium chloride, Calcium gluconate* and Oral Rehydration Salt (ORS), Physiological acid base balance.

- **Dental products:** Dentifrices, role of fluoride in the treatment of dental caries, Desensitizing agents, Calcium carbonate, Sodium fluoride, and Zinc eugenol cement.

UNIT-III   10 Hours

- **Gastrointestinal agents**

Acidifiers: Ammonium chloride* and Dil. HCl

Antacid: Ideal properties of antacids, combinations of antacids, Sodium 40 Bicarbonate*, Aluminum hydroxide gel, Magnesium hydroxide mixture

Cathartics: Magnesium sulphate, Sodium orthophosphate, Kaolin and Bentonite

Antimicrobials: Mechanism, classification, Potassium permanganate, Boric acid, Hydrogen peroxide*, Chlorinated lime*, Iodine and its preparations

UNIT-IV   08 Hours

- **Miscellaneous compounds:**

Expectorants: Potassium iodide, Ammonium chloride*.

Emetics: Copper sulphate*, Sodium potassium tartarate

Haematinics: Ferrous sulphate*, Ferrous gluconate

Poison and Antidote: Sodium thiosulphate*, Activated charcoal, Sodium nitrite333

Astringents: Zinc Sulphate, Potash Alum

UNIT-V

- **Radiopharmaceuticals:** Radio activity, Measurement of radioactivity, Properties of α, β, γ radiations, Half-life, radio isotopes and study of radio isotopes - Sodium iodide I^{131} , Storage conditions, precautions & pharmaceutical application of radioactive substances.

UNIT – 1
IMPURITIES IN PHARMACEUTICAL SUBSTANCES

Q.1. Define Pharmacopoeia with an example?

For preparation of medicines there is a requirement of specific directions which are written in a book known as Pharmacopoeia. Usually, a pharmacopoeia is published by a concerned authority, and is established by the government. Therefore, pharmacopoeia is a legislation of a country responsible for setting standards as well as parameters related to quality and quantity of drugs, and raw materials required for the preparation of several pharmaceutical formulations.

Pharmacopoeia is a collection of drugs and therapeutic substances with directions and methods for preparation. Pharmacopoeia means a book of standards applicable to drugs and their common dosage forms and pharmaceutical aids published in a country under the authority of its own government.

Most of the advanced countries have their own Pharmacopoeias. **For example,** Indian Pharmacopoeia (I.P.) and British Pharmacopoeia (B.P.) are published under the authority of respective governments. The first British was published in the year 1864 and many editions of this book have published since then. United States Pharmacopoeia (U.S.P.) published in U.S.A. is another important book in this regard.

Q.2.What is a Pharmacopoeia? Give I.P a quick note.

Pharmacopoeia: Pharmacopoeia is a collection of drugs and therapeutic substances with directions and methods for preparation. Pharmacopoeia means a book of standards applicable to drugs and their common dosage forms and pharmaceutical aids published in a country under the authority of its own government. For preparation of medicines there is a requirement of specific directions which are written in a book known as **Pharmacopoeia**. Most of the advanced countries have their own Pharmacopoeias.

For example, Indian Pharmacopoeia (I.P.) and British Pharmacopoeia (B.P.) are published under the authority of respective governments.

Indian Pharmacopoeia (I.P.): Indian Pharmacopoeia (I.P.) is an official document meant for overall quality control and assurance of pharmaceutical products marketed in India by way of contributing on their safety, efficacy, and affordability. I.P. contains a collection of standard procedures of analysis and specifications for drugs. The I.P. or any part of it, has got legal status under the Second Schedule of the Drugs & Cosmetics Act, 1940 and Rules 1945 thereunder.

I.P. prescribes standards for identity, purity, and strength of drugs essentially required from healthcare perspective of human beings and animals. I.P. standards are authoritative in nature. They are enforced by the Regulatory Authorities for quality control of medicines in India. During quality assurance and at the time of dispute in the court of law, the LP. standards are legally acceptable.

The Indian Pharmacopoeia is published by the Indian Pharmacopoeia Commission (IPC) on behalf of the Ministry of Health and Family Welfare, Government of India. The Indian Pharmacopoeia is being prepared to fulfil the requirements in the Drugs and Cosmetics Rules, 1945 of standards of drugs produced in India and in the belief that it contributes significantly in controlling the quality of medicinal products. The standards of this pharmacopoeia are legally enforceable and are intended to help in the licensing and inspection processes.

Q.3. Write a detailed note on Indian Pharmacopoeia.

Indian Pharmacopoeia (I.P.):

➢ Indian Pharmacopoeia (I.P.) is an official document meant for overall quality control and assurance of pharmaceutical products marketed in India by way of contributing on their safety, efficacy, and affordability.

➢ I.P. contains a collection of standard procedures of analysis and specifications for drugs.

➢ The I.P. or any part of it, has got legal status under the Second Schedule of the Drugs & Cosmetics Act, 1940 and Rules 1945 thereunder.

➢ I.P. prescribes standards for identity, purity, and strength of drugs essentially required from healthcare perspective of human beings and animals.

➢ I.P. standards are authoritative in nature. They are enforced by the Regulatory Authorities for quality control of medicines in India.

- During quality assurance and at the time of dispute in the court of law, the LP. standards are legally acceptable.
- The Indian Pharmacopoeia is published by the Indian Pharmacopoeia Commission (IPC) on behalf of the Ministry of Health and Family Welfare, Government of India.
- The Indian Pharmacopoeia is being prepared to fulfil the requirements in the Drugs and Cosmetics Rules, 1945 of standards of drugs produced in India and in the belief that it contributes significantly in controlling the quality of medicinal products.
- The standards of this pharmacopoeia are legally enforceable and are intended to help in the licensing and inspection processes.
- **The Indian Pharmacopoeia editions are as follows:**

1. Indian Pharmacopoeia 1955: First edition, followed by its supplement in 1960,
2. Indian Pharmacopoeia 1966: Second edition, followed by its supplement in 1975,
3. Indian Pharmacopoeia 1985: Third edition, followed by its addendum in 1989 and 1991,
4. Indian Pharmacopoeia 1996: Fourth edition, followed by its addendum in 2000 and 2002,
5. Indian Pharmacopoeia 2007: Fifth edition, followed by its addendum in 2008,
6. Indian 2010: Sixth edition, followed by its addendum in 2012; and DVD of Indian Pharmacopoeia 2010, and

7. Indian Pharmacopoeia 2014 with DVD: Seventh edition, followed by its addendum in 2015.

Q.4. Give a brief note on the history of pharmacopeia

Pharmacopeia: Pharmacopeia is derived from the Greek word **'Pharmakon'** mean **Drug** and **'Poiea'** mean **to make**. It is a legal and official book issued by recognized authorities usually appointed by the **Government of each country**. It compares a list of pharmaceutical substances and formulae along with their description and standards.

A drug included in pharmacopeia is termed official and sections dealing with official drugs preparation and substances are known as monographs.

History of Pharmacopeia: The history of I.P. began in the year 1833 when a committee of the East Indian Company's Dispensary recommended the publication of a Pharmacopoeia and Bengal Pharmacopoeia. The General Conspectus of Medicinal Plants was published in 1844, which mainly listed most commonly used indigenous remedies. This was followed by I.P. 1868, which covered both the drugs of British Pharmacopoeia (B.P.) 1867 and indigenous drugs used in India, with a supplement published in 1869 incorporating the vernacular names of indigenous drugs and plants.

However, from 1885 the B.P. was made official in India. A Drug Enquiry Committee appointed in 1927 by the government recommended the publication of a National Pharmacopoeia.

After independence, in year 1948 the Indian Pharmacopoeia Committee was constituted with a goal to publish an Indian Pharmacopoeia.

The **Indian Pharmacopoeia editions** are as follows:

1. **Indian Pharmacopoeia 1955:** First edition, followed by its supplement in 1960,

2. **Indian Pharmacopoeia 1966:** Second edition, followed by its supplement in 1975,

3. **Indian Pharmacopoeia 1985:** Third edition, followed by its addendum in 1989 and 1991,

4. **Indian Pharmacopoeia 1996:** Fourth edition, followed by its addendum in 2000 and 2002,

5. **Indian Pharmacopoeia 2007:** Fifth edition, followed by its addendum in 2008,

6. **Indian 2010:** Sixth edition, followed by its addendum in 2012; and DVD of Indian Pharmacopoeia 2010, and 7) Indian Pharmacopoeia 2014 with DVD: Seventh edition, followed by its addendum in 2015.

Q.5. Give a brief note on the development of pharmacopeia.

Pharmacopeia: Pharmacopeia is derived from the Greek word **'Pharmakon'** mean **Drug** and **'Poiea'** mean **to make**. It is a legal and official book issued by recognized authorities usually appointed by the **Government of each country**. It comparises a list of pharmaceutical substances and formulae along with their description and standards.

A drug included in pharmacopoeia is termed official and sections dealing with official drugs preparation and substances are known as monographs.

development of pharmacopeia: In the year **1948**, Indian Pharmacopoeia Committee was formed which published the **Pharmacopoeia of India** (The Indian Pharmacopoeia) in the year **1955**, while its supplement was published in the year 1960. Western as well as traditional drugs were included in the **1st edition**, while same pattern was followed in the **2nd edition** of India Pharmacopoeia which was published in the year **1966** and its supplement in **1975**.

The **3rd edition** of Indian Pharmacopoeia was published in the year **1985** and its addendum in the year **1989** and **1991**. This edition included only those herbal drugs which have specific parameters for their quality control, while other traditional drugs were not included in this pharmacopoeia, but published separately.

The 3rd edition significantly increased the range of drug products. This led to addition or deletion of many monographs by the Committee as per the priorities of drugs used and their medical merit in the **4th edition** which was published in the year **1996**. Its addendum was published in the years **2000, 2002**, and **2005**. Along with all these a supplement was also published in the year **2002** which contains a list of veterinary products.

The **5ᵗʰ edition** of Indian Pharmacopoeia was published in the year **2007**. whereas its addendum was published in the year **2008**. This edition was prepared according to the principles and plans which were designed by a scientific body of Indian Pharmacopoeia Commission. The monographs, general notices, testing methods, etc., were based on advanced technology and experimental methods which are adopted both nationally and internationally. The appendices are, amended according to the methods employed for monitoring the quality of drugs internationally. Special relevance is given to the monographs related to the medicines used for endemic diseases.

The **Indian Pharmacopoeia, 2007** is presented in the following three volumes:

1. **Volume 1** contains the general notices, preface, and structure of the I.P.C., acknowledgement, introduction, and the general chapters.
2. **Volume 2** deals with the general monographs on the drugs substances, dosage forms, and pharmaceutical aids (A-M).
3. **Volume 3** contains monographs on drug substances, dosage forms and pharmaceutical aids (N-Z) followed by monographs on vaccines an immunizer for human use, herbs and herbal products, blood and blood related products, biotechnology products, and veterinary products.

The **6ᵗʰ edition** of Indian Pharmacopoeia was published in the year **2010** and contains three volumes:

1. **Volume I** consist of notices, preface, constituents of I.P.C., acknowledgements, introduction, and general chapters.

2. **Volume II** consist of general notices, general monographs related to dosage forms, monographs related to drug substances, dosage forms, and pharmaceutical aids from alphabet A-M.

3. **Volume III** consist of monographs related to drug substances, dosage forms, and pharmaceutical aids from alphabet N-Z. This volume also contains monographs of vaccines and immunosera used by humans, herbs and herbal products, blood and products related to blood, products related to biotechnology and veterinary.

Salient Features of I.P. Sixth Edition: It comprises of some special characteristics such as:

1. It is available in three volumes which are hard bound.

2. It contains a total of 1918 monographs, out of which 287 were newly added.

3. Categorization, dosage, and available strength of dose for the drug were also added.

4. Traditional tests were replaced by more specific tests, such as IR and UV spectrophotometry.

5. Cross referencing was also eliminated.

6. Presentation of the subject matter is in more uniform manner.

7. Application of chromatography is done extensively.

8. Pyrogen testing was also eliminated up to certain limits.

9. Monographs related to herbal drugs are also added.

10. It also contains many monographs which are not present in other major pharmacopoeias globally.

11. It also contains a certificate to prove its authenticity

12. The format is quite simple and easy to understand.

The **latest edition** of the Indian Pharmacopoeia is the **7th edition** and was published in **2014** by the **Indian Pharmacopoeia Commission** (I.P.C.) for the Ministry of Health and Family Welfare, Government of India.

The publishing of Indian Pharmacopoeia, 2014 was done according to the principles and plans designed and decided by the scientific body of the Indian Pharmacopoeia Commission. The monographs, appendices, as well as other revised information are made public on the website of I.P.C. It was done in order to gain transparency in setting standards as well as for getting feedback from the public. These feedbacks are reviewed by the expert members of the committee for testing viability and practicality of methods and standards. At the time of the compilation of Indian Pharmacopoeia 2014 edition, the principle of **'openness, justice,** and **fairness'** were also considered.

The Indian Pharmacopoeia 2014 is presented in four volumes. The scope of the pharmacopoeia has been extended after including additional anticancer drugs and antiretroviral drugs and formulations, products of biotechnology. indigenous herbs and herbal products, and veterinary vaccines.

Standards for new drugs and drugs used under National Health Programs are added and the drugs as well as their formulations which are not in use nowadays are omitted from this edition.

The I.P. 2014 incorporates **2548 monographs of drugs**, out of which **577 are new monographs** consisting of APIs, excipients, dosage forms, herbal products, etc. It is hoped that this edition would play a significant role in improving the quality of medicines, which in turn promote public health and accelerate the growth and development of Pharma Sector.

Salient Features of I.P. 7th Edition: The I.P. 2014 was scheduled to be effective from 1st January, 2014, but came into effect from **1st April, 2014**. The reason behind the delay was to give the much-needed time to industries so as to adopt the changes and policies under the I.P. 2014. The **features of the 7th edition I.P. 2014** includes:

1. A total of 2548 monographs were added.
2. This edition also contains 577 new monographs.
3. 19 monographs and 1 general chapter were added related to radiopharmaceuticals.
4. The edition comprises of 4 volumes which are available in hard bound along with a DVD.
5. Cross referencing was eliminated.
6. The monographs related to veterinary are considered to be vital portion of this edition.
7. A uniform pattern is followed for presenting the subject matter.

8. The use of chromatographic methods is extensively mentioned.

9. Traditional tests were replaced by more specific tests, such as IR UV spectrophotometry.

10. Pyrogen testing was eliminated virtually.

11. Monographs which were irrelevant were eliminated.

12. Many monographs related to herbs were added.

13. It also contains many monographs which are not present in other pharmacopoeias globally.

14. It also contains a certificate to prove its authenticity.

15. The format is quite easy and simple to understand.

Q.6. Give a short note on the latest edition of pharmacopeia.

Latest Edition- 7ᵗʰ Edition of Indian Pharmacopoeia, 2014: The **latest edition** of the Indian Pharmacopoeia is the **7th edition** and was published in **2014** by the **Indian Pharmacopoeia Commission** (I.P.C.) for the Ministry of Health and Family Welfare, Government of India.

The publishing of Indian Pharmacopoeia, 2014 was done according to the principles and plans designed and decided by the scientific body of the Indian Pharmacopoeia Commission. The monographs, appendices, as well as other revised information are made public on the website of I.P.C. It was done in order to gain transparency in setting standards as well as for getting feedback from the public. These feedbacks are reviewed by the expert members of the committee for testing viability and practicality of methods and standards. At the time of compilation of Indian Pharmacopoeia 2014 edition, the principle of **'openness, justice,** and **fairness'** were also considered.

The Indian Pharmacopoeia 2014 is presented in four volumes. The scope of the pharmacopoeia has been extended after including additional anticancer drugs and antiretroviral drugs and formulations, products of biotechnology. indigenous herbs and herbal products, and veterinary vaccines.

Standards for new drugs and drugs used under National Health Programs are added and the drugs as well as their formulations which are not in use nowadays are omitted from this edition.

The I.P. 2014 incorporates **2548 monographs of drugs**, out of which **577are new monographs** consisting of APIs, excipients, dosage forms, herbal products, etc. It is hoped that this edition would play a significant role in improving the quality of medicines, which in turn promote public health and accelerate the growth and development of Pharma Sector.

Salient Features of I.P. 7th Edition: The I.P. 2014 was scheduled to be effective from 1st January, 2014, but came into effect from **1st April, 2014**. The reason behind the delay was to give much-needed time to industries so as to adopt the changes and policies under the I.P. 2014. The **features of the 7th edition I.P. 2014** includes:

1. A total of 2548 monographs were added.
2. This edition also contains 577 new monographs.

3. 19 monographs and 1 general chapter were added related to radiopharmaceuticals.

4. The edition comprises of 4 volumes which are available in hard bound along with a DVD.

5. Cross referencing was eliminated.

6. The monographs related to veterinary are considered to be vital portion of this edition.

7. A uniform pattern is followed for presenting the subject matter.

8. The use of chromatographic methods is extensively mentioned.

9. Traditional tests were replaced by more specific tests, such as IR UV spectrophotometry.

10. Pyrogen testing was eliminated virtually.

11. Monographs which were irrelevant were eliminated.

12. Many monographs related to herbs were added.

13. It also contains many monographs which are not present in other pharmacopoeias globally.

14. It also contains a certificate to prove its authenticity.

15. The format is quite easy and simple to understand.

Q.7. Give salient features of the latest edition of I.P.

The **latest edition** of the Indian Pharmacopoeia is the **7th edition** and was published in **2014** by the **Indian Pharmacopoeia Commission** (I.P.C.) for the Ministry of Health and Family Welfare, Government of India.

The publishing of Indian Pharmacopoeia, 2014 was done according to the principles and plans designed and decided by the scientific body of the Indian Pharmacopoeia Commission.

The monographs, appendices, as well as other revised information, are made public on the website of I.P.C.

Salient Features of I.P. 7th Edition: The I.P. 2014 was scheduled to be effective from 1st January, 2014, but came into effect from **1st April, 2014**. The reason behind the delay was to give the much-needed time to industries so as to adopt the changes and policies under the I.P. 2014. The **features of the 7th edition I.P. 2014** includes:

1. A total of 2548 monographs were added.
2. This edition also contains 577 new monographs.
3. 19 monographs and 1 general chapter were added related to radiopharmaceuticals.
4. The edition comprises of 4 volumes which are available in hard bound along with a DVD.
5. Cross referencing was eliminated.
6. The monographs related to veterinary are considered to be vital portion of this edition.
7. A uniform pattern is followed for presenting the subject matter.
8. The use of chromatographic methods is extensively mentioned.
9. Traditional tests were replaced by more specific tests, such as IR UV spectrophotometry.

10. Pyrogen testing was eliminated virtually.

11. Monographs which were irrelevant were eliminated.

12. Many monographs related to herbs were added.

13. It also contains many monographs which are not present in other pharmacopoeias globally.

14. It also contains a certificate to prove its authenticity.

15. The format is quite easy and simple to understand.

Q.8. Define Impurities. Enlist the sources of the impurities in Pharmaceuticals and discuss the manufacturing hazards as a source of impurity.

Impurities: The presence of foreign matter or impurities makes a compound impure. Therefore, impurities can be defined as substances present within a limited quantity of solid, liquid, or gas. Impurities also differ from the compound in which they are present with respect to their chemical composition.

Generally, the level of impurities in a compound is defined relatively, by comparing test material with the standard one. Impurities may occur either naturally in a compound or may be added deliberately, accidentally, inevitably, or incidentally during the manufacturing of the product.

List the sources of impurities:

1. Raw materials employed in manufacture
2. Reagents used in the manufacturing process
3. Processes used in the manufacture

4. Environment related impurities
5. Defects in manufacturing process
6. Manufacturing hazards
7. Impurities arising during storage
8. Accidental substitution or deliberate adulteration with spurious

Manufacturing Hazards: While manufacturing a product, following types of contamination may occur:

i) Particulate Contamination: Accidental access of dirt, glass, porcelain, metallic or plastic fragments from sieves, granulating. tableting and filling machines or from product containers are the various sources give rise to the contaminants. **For example**, eye ointments packed in metal tubes (aluminium and tin) consist of traces of metal particles. Metal splinters are produced during the manufacturing process of the tube. Although, these metal particulates are not easy to remove from the inner lining of the tube, even by washing and cleaning, some of them are excluded along with the ointment, thus, enhancing its viscosity. However, the particulates produced by tin are larger than that of aluminium.

ii) Process Errors (Gross Errors): Incomplete solution of a solute in a liquid formulation rise to gross errors. Normal analytical techniques are used for detecting such errors. While preparing such solutions, some precautions should be taken. One of the precautions that can be taken is filtering the solution which prevents the contamination of the product by the un-dissolved solute.

iii) Cross Contamination: A huge quantity of air-borne dust is released during the handling of large bulk of powders, granules, and tablets. The so released dust particles can contaminate the final product, if preventive measures are not taken. Cross contamination can be prevented by using face masks and special equipment for extraction.

iv) Microbial Contamination: The sterility tests for parenteral and ophthalmic preparations provide an adequate level of control. regardless of their preparation by end sterilisation process or under septic conditions. Other formulations which are prone to bacterial mould and fungal contamination or equipment contamination during their manufacturing are liquid preparations or equipment and creams for topical application over broken skin or mucous membranes.

v) Packing Errors: Mislabelling may occur of either one or both the drugs similar in appearance, such as tablets of the same size, colour and shape and packed in similar containers. Such similar products should not be handled together and to avoid such accidents control measures should be taken.

Q.9. Write sources oof impurities in pharmaceutical substances.

Source of Impurities in pharmaceutical substances: The impurities in drug products may be obtained from various sources which are same for the reference drug products also. Starting materials, by-products, residual solvents, chemical degrades formed and long-term storage are the main sources of impurities. Heat, light, changing pH, interaction with packaging materials and other components also results in impurities.

The most common sources of impurities are:

1. Raw Materials Employed in Manufacture: Impurities resulting from raw materials may affect the process of manufacture and contaminate the resultant product. **For example**, traces of calcium sulphate and magnesium chloride are present in rock salt so that a small quantity of calcium and magnesium will be present in the sodium chloride produced from this.

The impurities (**like arsenic, lead, heavy metals**, etc.) present in raw materials may get transfer to the end product, therefore, it is essential to purify the raw material or starting chemicals. For example, bismuth compounds show traces of lead, copper, and silver obtained from the raw materials used for their production.

The impurity type that a substance may contain also depends manufacturing process. **For example**, action of sulphuric acid copper turnings produces copper sulphate

$$Cu + 2H_2SO_4 \rightarrow CuSO_4 + 2H_2O + SO_4$$

Iron and arsenic may be present in copper turnings in the form of impurities, either in small or in large quantity. These impurities may contaminate the final product, i.e., CuSO4.5H2O, if raw materials contain them in large quantity.

2. Reagents Used in the Manufacturing Process: The impurities from the reagents may contaminate the final product, if they are not washed away properly. **For example**, mixing mercuric chloride solution with dilute ammonia solution results in ammoniated mercury:

$$HgCl_2 + NH_4OH \rightarrow NH_2HgCl + NH_4Cl + 2H_2O$$

The ammonium hydroxide present in the final product, i.e., the ammoniated mercury precipitate, can be removed by washing away with cold water. If not eliminated by washing, it may remain in the product as an impurity.

3. Processes Used in Manufacture: Different manufacturing processes are used for producing many drugs and chemicals (especially organic). During these processes of manufacturing some impurities get an access into the materials. However, the drugs or chemicals may contain varying kind and quantity of impurities. For some drugs, a multiple-step synthesis procedure is used for the production of intermediate compounds. These intermediate compounds need to be purified to reduce the contamination of final product. Synthesis of the intermediate compounds is mainly brought about by side reactions. The impurities present in the resultant product of these side reactions are also found in the substances.

Due to the adulteration caused by reagents and solvents, following impurities may access the final product at various stages of reaction:

i) Formulation Related Impurities: Most of the impurities found in a drug product are produced from excipients. During the formulation, the drug goes through various reactions, resulting in its degradation and detrimental reactions. **For example**, a product may degrade if it is dried by heating. Another example is that the solutions or suspensions are more likely to degrade due to hydrolysis or solvolysis.

ii) Synthetic Intermediates and By-Products: Raw materials, solvents, intermediates and by-products are the most common sources of impurities that enter the pharmaceutical preparations during synthesis. A drug substance is manufactured much more purity requirements than the raw material. The appreciable quantity of solvents used during synthesis cannot be neglected, as these impurities may further undergo reaction chemicals and produce major impurities in the synthetic reaction.

iii) Residual Solvents: During manufacturing residual solvents (organic or inorganic liquids) are used and their complete eradication is difficult. For manufacturing bulk drugs, toxic solvents should not be used. The **residual solvents are categorised into three classes** depending upon the risk it possesses towards the human health:

a) Class I: Solvents like benzene and carbon tetrachloride with 2ppm and 4ppm limit, respectively.

b) Class II: Methylene chloride (600ppm limit), methanol (3000ppm limit), pyridine (200ppm limit), toluene (890ppmlimit), and acetonitrile (410ppm limit).

c) Class III: Acetic acid, acetone, isopropyl alcohol, butanol, ethanol and ethyl acetate have permitted daily exposures of 50mg or less per day.

iv) Method Related Impurities: During formulation, due to exposure to heat, light, pH change, solvents, etc., impurities are produced, **e.g.,** autoclaving of diclofenac sodium generates 1-(2,6-dichlorophenyl)-indolin-2-one.

v) Chemical Processes Used in Manufacture: Nitration, halogenation, oxidation, reduction, hydrolysis etc., are the various reactions involved in the synthesis of drugs.

These chemical reactions make use of various chemicals. **For example,** potassium iodide is manufactured from iodine, obtained from kelp; when nitrogenous organic matter and alkalis are burned together, sea weed cyanides are formed.

4. Environment Related Impurities: Atmosphere in industrial areas is adulterated with some gases like hydrogen sulphide, sulphur dioxide and black smoke (soot), and dust particles (aluminium oxide, silica glass particles, porcelain particles, plastic fragments, etc.). These impurities contaminate the final product during the manufacturing and purification of pharmaceutical preparations.

Following are the environmental factors which impure the drug substances:

i) Exposure to Adverse Temperature: Many drug substances are sensitive to heat or tropical temperature, **for example**, vitamins are thermolabile, therefore their potency is decreased.

ii) UV Light: Ergometrine and methyl ergometrine injection are unstable under tropical conditions (such as light and heat). As per the report of several studies, very low active ingredient is found in ergometrine and methyl ergometrine injection under these conditions.

iii) Humidity: Bulk powder and formulated solid dosage forms (like, aspirin and ranitidine) may get affected by humidity due to their hygroscopic nature.

5. Defects in Manufacturing Process: Defects like imperfect mixing, incompleteness, non-adherence to proper temperature, pressure, pH or reaction conditions, etc., generate impurities during the manufacturing of chemical compounds. **For example**, adding pure calcium carbonate to excess of dilute hydrochloric acid, followed by stirring and filtration results in the production of calcium chloride ($CaCl_2.6H_2O$). On further concentrating the filtrate, crystals of $CaCl_2.6H_2O$ are produced.

$$CaCO_3 + 2HCl \rightarrow CaCl_2 + H_2O + CO_2$$

Slight excess of calcium carbonate is added with the objective to consume hydrochloric acid which may enter the filtrate. Some amount of unreacted HCl remains in the solution, if it is not properly mixed with $CaCO_3$. This unreacted HCl enters the filtrate and penetrates the

$CaCl_2.6H_2O$ crystals. Therefore, to check the presence or absence of acid in $CaCl_2.6H_2O$, an acidity test has been prescribed by the I.P.

6. Manufacturing Hazards: While manufacturing a product, following types of contamination may occur:

i) Particulate Contamination: Accidental access of dirt, glass, porcelain, metallic or plastic fragments from sieves, granulating. tableting and filling machines or from product containers are the various sources give rise to the contaminants. **For example**, eye ointments packed in metal tubes (aluminium and tin) consist of traces of metal particles. Metal splinters are produced during the manufacturing process of the tube. Although, these metal particulates are not easy to remove from the inner lining of the tube, even by washing and cleaning, some of them are excluded along with the ointment, thus, enhancing its viscosity. However, the particulates produced by tin are larger than that of aluminium.

ii) Process Errors (Gross Errors): Incomplete solution of a solute in a liquid formulation rise to gross errors. Normal analytical techniques are used for detecting such errors. While preparing such solutions, some precautions should be taken. One of the precautions that can be taken is filtering the solution which prevents the contamination of the product by the un-dissolved solute.

iii) Cross Contamination: A huge quantity of air-borne dust is released during the handling of large bulk of powders, granules, and tablets. The so released dust particles can contaminate the final product, if preventive measures are not taken. Cross contamination can be prevented by using face masks and special equipment for extraction.

iv) Microbial Contamination: The sterility tests for parenteral and ophthalmic preparations provide an adequate level of control. regardless of their preparation by end sterilisation process or under septic conditions. Other formulations which are prone to bacterial mould and fungal contamination or equipment contamination during their manufacturing are liquid preparations or equipment and creams for topical application over broken skin or mucous membranes.

v) Packing Errors: Mislabelling may occur of either one or both the drugs similar in appearance, such as tablets of the same size, colour and shape and packed in similar containers. Such similar products should not be handled together and to avoid such accidents control measures should be taken.

7. Impurities Arising During Storage: After the preparation of different chemicals and substances, they need to be stored in containers. The type of containers required for storage are available in a variety (such as plastic, polythene, iron vessels, stainless steel, aluminium, copper, etc.) and depends upon the factors, 'like material's nature, batch size, and quantity. The interaction between the stored substances and the storage container's material give rise to impurities.

Following are the inefficient storage conditions and their effects:

i) Filth: If preventive measures are not taken, dust, insect bodies, animal and insect excreta may pollute the stored products. All these contaminations can be removed from the final products by using modern techniques of packaging. However, raw materials stored in bulk (vegetable drugs) give rise to such adulteration. Thus, all the stored materials should be tested to confirm the presence or absence of filth.

ii) Chemical Instability: This is another cause of contamination of the stored products. If pharmaceutical preparations are stored in inappropriate storage conditions, they undergo chemical decomposition. The chemical decomposition may also be catalysed by light, acid or alkali, oxidation, water vapour, carbon dioxide, or metallic ions. The chemical properties of the substance help in determining the nature of decomposition the product undergoes.

Use of antioxidants, like phenols (including Butylated hydroxy anisole, Butylated hydroxytoluene and thymol) prevents oxidation as they undergo free radical oxidation instead of the substance (**e.g.,** liquid paraffin) they are intended to protect.

Another antioxidant used is sodium metabisulphite which undergoes oxidation and gets converted to sodium bisulphate. This antioxidant is best suited for aqueous solution (**e.g.,** procaine and adrenaline injection).

iii) Reaction with Container Materials: The reaction between the container and its contents may be hazardous. To avoid such hazards, metal tubes should not be used for packaging ointments which are likely to react with metal (**e.g.**, salicylic acid ointment).

However, metal tubes can be used if their internal surface has been lacquered to prevent reaction. Glass ampoules should be used for packing solutions of alkali sensitive materials, if they have undergone heat treatment while being prepared (**e.g.**, atropine sulphate injection sterilised by autoclaving).

iv) Physical Changes: These changes occurring in the stored drug are well known. The product efficiency is highly affected due to the changes in crystal size and form, agglomeration and caking of suspended particles. Therefore, the absorption rate and bioavailability of low solubility drugs (e.g., griseofulvin) can be determined by the particle size and surface area.

v) Temperature: Temperature affects the rate at which a stored product undergoes chemical and physical changes. In order to prevent decomposition, special storage conditions are maintained for temperature sensitive materials. Instructions, like "store in a cool place" are clearly interpreted by the operator.

8. Accidental Substitution or Deliberate Adulteration with Spurious or Useless Materials: By separately stocking all the toxic substances together or in a locked cupboard, accidental substitution can be prevented. Materials should be purchased carefully since most of the time adulteration is done intentionally as a result of inefficient enforcement of Drugs and Cosmetics Act.

Many pharmaceutical chemicals are adulterated with cheap substances, **e.g.**, expensive KBr is adulterated with cheaper NaBr. Therefore, a test for sodium has been prescribed by the I.P. to prevent KBr from getting adulterated. Therefore, those substances which can be analytically controlled can be used to adulterate crude drugs, essential oils, fats, and other substances.

Q.10. Discuss types of impurities in pharmaceutical substances.

Impurities in Pharmaceutical Substances: Presence of foreign matter or impurities makes a compound impure. Therefore, impurities can be defined as substances present within a limited quantity of solid, liquid, or gas. Impurities also differ from the compound in which they are present with respect to their chemical composition.

Generally, level of impurities in a compound is defined relatively, by comparing test material with the standard one. Impurities may occur either naturally in a compound or may be added deliberately, accidentally, inevitably, or incidentally during the manufacturing of the product.

Types of Impurities: Impurities are categorized into two types depending upon the effect they produce on the product:

1. **Destructive Impurities:** Impurities, like leaf pieces in blank white papers, ash and debris in metals, hinders the material's function, thus are said to be destructive.

   Such impurities can be removed from the material by employing **two methods**:

i. **Chemical Methods:** (Some impurities from a compound can be removed chemically. **For example**, calcium carbonate is added to the blast furnace while manufacturing iron to remove silicon dioxide from the iron ore Another method used is **zone refining** which is economically advantageous and is used for purifying semi-conductors.

ii. **Physical Methods:** Some impurities can also be removed by using physical methods. **For example**, by using distillation method, water and salt mixture can be separated. In this method, water is employed as a distillate and salt as the solid residue. By utilizing physical means, liquids, gases, metal ore, etc. can also be freed from the impurities.

2. **Constructive Impurities:** Some impurities prove to be useful for a compound, thus, are said to be constructive. **For example**, metals and impurities are combined form alloys. This combination has properties which are more desirable than the constituent materials.

Another example is adding less than 2% of carbon in pure iron to manufacture steel. Another method of employing constructive impurities is **doping of silicon**. This method involves mixing of 0.001-0.01% impurities with silicon the form of phosphorus and boron atoms during the production of solar cells. This addition of phosphorus and boron (which can be called as impurities) helps in generating electricity.

Q.11. Write a short note on pharmaceutical impurities.

Pharmaceutical Impurities: Different types of impurities, like raw materials, dust particles, moisture," etc. may be present in the chemical compounds manufactured commercially. However, the total quantity of these impurities is small.

Pharmaceutical products may contain the following impurities:

1. **Toxic impurities, e.g.,** lead and arsenic salts.
2. **Activity depressing impurities, e.g.,** presence of water in hard soap.
3. **Impurities causing incompatibility** make a substance incompatible with other substance.
4. **Impurities causing technical difficulties, e.g.,** presence of potassium iodate (KIO3) in potassium iodide (KI) or presence of carbonate in ammonia solutions.
5. **Impurities due to coloring** or **flavoring** substances, **e.g.,** discoloration of sodium salicylate by phenolic compounds; dampness of sodium chloride in the presence of magnesium salts.
6. **Humidity or traces of moisture** reduces the free-flowing property of substances; thus, they may get easily oxidized.
7. **Impurities changing the physical and chemical properties** of the and making them undesirable for medicinal use.
8. **Impurities decreasing the shelf-life** of a compound.

Q.12. Write a detail note on Limit and effects of impurities present in pharmaceutical substances.

Limit: The process of acquiring and evaluating data that establishes a safety limit for an individual impurity or establishment of impurity profile at the level(s) not being harmful is the limit of impurities or qualification.

Applicants are recommended to provide a rationale for establishing impurity acceptance criteria that includes safety considerations.

If the following conditions are fulfilled by an impurity, it is considered to be qualified:

1. If the level considered and the criteria accepted for impurity does not exceed the level considered in FDA and is approved for human drug product,
2. If the impurity is a metabolite of the drug,
3. If the level observed and the criteria accepted for impurity is justified by the scientific literature in an efficient manner, and
4. If the level observed and the criteria accepted for impurity does not exceed the level evaluated properly in comparison to in vitro genotoxicity studies.

Effect: A little amount of impurity always remain in a material, therefore, preparing a completely pure substance is not only difficult but almost impossible.

Following effects may be produced by the impurities present in a substance:

1. If the level of toxic impurities exceeds a certain limit, it proves out to be injurious as therapeutic substances.

2. After a certain period, even minute quantity of impurities causes toxic effects.

3. Some impurities are useful if present in small quantity. But, if its quantity lowers the active strength of the substance, its therapeutic efficiency decreases.

4. Impurities alter the physical and chemical properties of a substance thus, making it therapeutically inactive.

5. Impurities also bring about technical difficulties in the formulation.

6. Some impurities result in incompatibility with other substances.

7. Impurities also reduce the shelf-life of a substance.

8. Some impurities do not cause any harmful effect but changes color, odour, taste, etc. of a substance, therefore, making the substance unhygienic and unfit to use.

Q.13. Give a detail note on Quality Control of impurity.

Quality Control of Impurities: Medicinal compounds should be of pure quality, devoid of unnecessary toxic and undesirable substances. A substance must be pure as much as possible, since, avoiding any impurity completely is a tedious task.

Regarding the problems caused by impurities in a substance, the pharmacopoeia committee considers the following points:

1. **Limits for Deleterious Impurities:** The deleterious impurities (lead and arsenic) should not be present in excessive

amounts. Therefore, limits for such impurities have been mentioned in the pharmacopoeias.

The substances also undergo tests to detect the presence of such impurities and to check whether or not the quantity of impurities present is within the prescribed limit.

2. **Limits for Harmless Impurities:** Pharmacopoeias have prescribed and fixed the limits for harmless impurities also, so that they do not alter the therapeutic efficacy of the drug.

    These limits depend on the factors, like nature of the impurity, type and use of the substance, etc. Harmful effects and incompatibilities produced by an impurity are considered while fixing the tolerance limit for a particular impurity.

    The impurities may also enhance the therapeutic efficacy of substances, in some cases. **For example**, copper traces enhance the therapeutic value of iron preparations, because it helps in the formation of hemoglobin (the purpose for which the iron preparations are usually administered) via catalytic activity.

3. **Cost:** Another point to be taken into account is attaining impurity free substances at moderate costs. Impurity free substances can be prepared by following a series of purification steps, but this is an over-priced method. Therefore, pharmacopoeias have prescribed the limits for various impurities.

4. **Adulteration:** Adulteration is adding a substance with similar qualities or adding impurities to the pure substance, **e.g.,**

sodium salt adulteration with potassium salt, magnesium salt adulteration with calcium salt, etc.

Although, adulterated substances also reflect therapeutic activity but ethical adulteration is legal. Therefore, pharmacopoeias fix limit for such impurities and also prescribe tests for their detection in the substances.

Q.14. What is Limit test? Write factor affecting of limit test.

Limit Test: Limit tests involve simple comparisons of opalescence, turbidity, or color with fixed standards.

Limit tests are **quantitative** or **semi quantitative** tests designed to identify & control small quantities of impurities which the substance is termed as **limit tests**.

Normally, an official preparation has only traces of impurity therefore, most of the time such preparations give negative results on carrying a limit test for impurity. In such a case, specialized or advanced test procedures should be adopted to avoid handling errors and to get better results.

Limit test is used for:

1. Finding out the quantity of **harmful impurity**, and
2. Finding out the quantity of **avoidable/unavoidable impurities**.

NOTE: In Performing limit tests only distilled water or purified water is used because ordinary tap water contains the number of ions to vitiate the test.

Factors affecting limit tests: The following factors are responsible for designing the various limit tests.

1. **Specificity of the tests:** Ideally a test is demanded which is very specific for the impurity present. Limit tests based on a thin layer, gas, and HPLC in which impurities are readily separated are useful techniques. The impurities peeves characteristics R_f values.

2. **Sensitivity:** The sensitivity of most texts is dependent upon a number of variable factors of the Precipitating reagent, duration of the reaction, and reaction temperature.
   Example: Cold dilute solution gives light precipitates.

3. **Control of Personal Errors**: The extent of the visible reaction should be clearly and precisely defined. The following ways if followed will control personal errors.
   a) **Test in which there is no visible reaction**: In this test, there is no color or precipitate, therefore it is very difficult to assess the presence of the impurity.
   b) **Comparison Methods**: This method can be effectively applied in many thin-layer chromatographic tests on a direct comparison with reference samples of impurities applied at a specific concentration.

c) **Quantitative determination**: It is only applied in special circumstances, usually where the limit is not readily susceptible to simple and more direct chemical determination. Loss on ignition, ash values, limits of moisture, Volatile matter, and residual solvents are some of the methods.

Q.15. Discuss the principle and reaction involved in the limit test of Chloride.

Limit Test for Chloride (I.P.): This test is carried out for identifying the chloride ions present in a standard solution.

Principle: Principle The limit test for chloride is based on a reaction that occurs between silver nitrate and soluble chlorides, resulting in silver chloride which is insoluble in dilute nitric acid.

$$Cl^- + AgNO_3 \xrightarrow{HNO_3} AgCl\downarrow + NO_3^-$$

The test solution appears turbid due to the formation of silver chloride in the presence of dilute nitric acid. Amount of chloride present in the test sample influences the degree of turbidity. The opalescent test solution is compared with a standard opalescent solution of known and acceptable limit. By viewing transversely through both the solutions against a black background in **Nessler's cylinder**, opalescence is compared. The sample passes the limit test, if the test solution is less turbid than the standard solution, and fails in vice versa condition.

Procedure: In this limit test, a standard solution and test solution is prepared and then the appearance of these two solutions is compared:

1. Test Solution: 1.0gm of sample is accurately weighed and transferred to Nessler cylinder A after dissolving in 10ml of distilled water. 1ml of nitric acid is added to this solution and volume is made up to 50ml with distilled water. 1ml of silver nitrate (5% w/v) is then added to the solution with stirring and the resultant solution is set aside for 5 minutes, after which turbidity develops.

2. Standard Solution: 1ml of 0.01N HCI is mixed with 1ml of nitric acid in Nessler cylinder B and volume is made up to 50ml with distilled water. Around 1ml of silver nitrate solution is then added which produces turbidity after 5 minutes or 1ml of 0.05845% w/v solution of sodium chloride is the standard source of chloride. The sample passes the limit test if it is less opalescent or turbid than the standard opalescence.

Test Solution	Standard Solution
Specified substance (1g) +10ml of water + 1ml of HNO_3	1ml of 0.05845% w/v solution of sodium chloride) + 1ml of HNO_3
Diluted to 50ml in Nessler cylinder Diluted to 50ml in **Nessler cylinder A**+ 1ml of $AgNO_3$ Solution	Diluted to 50ml in Nessler cylinder Diluted to 50ml in **Nessler cylinder B**+ 1ml of $AgNO_3$ Solution
Opalescence/turbidity	Opalescence/turbidity

Q.16. Discuss the principle and reaction involved in the limit test of Sulphate.

Limit Test for Sulphate (I.P. 1996): This test is carried out for controlling the sulphate impurity in inorganic

Principle: In this test, barium chloride reacts with soluble sulphate in the presence of dilute HCl solution. The resulting turbid solution is compared with the standard solution of acceptable limit. The barium sulphate reagent contains barium chloride, sulphate-free alcohol, and potassium sulphate. Alcohol prevents super-saturation, so the resulting turbidity is more uniform and potassium sulphate increases the sensitivity of test. The test solution fails to pass the test, if it develops more turbidity as compared to the standard solution.

$$SO_4^{2-} + BaCl_2 \rightarrow BaSO_4\downarrow + 2Cl^-$$

Procedure: In this limit test, a standard solution and test solution is prepared and then the appearance of these two solutions is compared:

1. Test Solution: 1gm of sulphate is weighed and 2ml of HCl is added to 45ml of solution. Then 5ml of $BaSO_4$ reagent is added to prepare the solution.

2. Standard Solution: 1ml of 0.1089% w/v solution of K_2SO_4 is weighed and treated with 2ml of HCl. This solution is diluted up to 45ml. At last the standard solution is prepared by adding 5ml of $BaSO_4$ reagent.

3. Barium Sulphate Reagent: 15ml of 0.5M barium chloride (122.1g/1000ml) is mixed with 55ml of water, 20ml of sulphate-free alcohol and 5ml of 0.0181% w/v solution of potassium sulphate. The resultant solution is diluted up to 100ml with water.

The test solution passes the limit test, if on observing it transversely against a black background it appears less opalescent than the standard solution.

Test Solution	Standard Solution
Specified substance (1g) + 2ml HCl diluted to 45ml + 5ml of $BaSO_4$ reagent	1ml of 0.1089% w/v solution of K_2SO_4 + 2ml HCl + H_2O dilute to 45ml + 5ml solution of $BaSO_4$ reagent
Turbidity	Turbidity

Q.17. Discuss the principle and reaction involved in the limit test of Iron.

Limit Test of Iron (L.P. 1996): This test is carried out for controlling the iron impurity in inorganic substances.

Principle: The limit test for iron relies on the reaction in which iron reacts with marcato acetic acid (thioglycolic acid) in a solution with ammonium citrate buffer. It results in the formation of a purple color solution due to the formation of ferrous mercaptoacetate (a coordination compound) and ferric iron being reduced to the ferrous state by the reagent. This purple color is compared with the standard color, containing a known amount of iron.

$$2\ Fe^{+++} + 2HS-CH_2COOH \rightarrow \begin{array}{c} S-CH_2-COOH \\ | \\ S-CH_2-COOH \end{array} + 2Fe^{++} + 2H^+$$

Ferric ion   Thioglycollic acid

$$Fe^{++} + 2HS-CH_2COOH \rightarrow \begin{array}{c} CH_2-COO \quad\quad SH \\ | \quad\quad\quad | \\ HS \quad\quad OOC-CH_2 \end{array} Fe + 2H^+$$

Fe^{++} Ferrous ion   Thioglycollic acid

Ferrous Thioglycollate complex
(purple colour)

Procedure: In this limit test, a standard and test solution is prepared, and the appearance of these two solutions is compared:

1. Test Solution: 40ml of water is added to the sample and treated with 2ml of 20% w/v citric acid. Then 2 drops of thioglycolic acid is added, the solution is mixed, made alkaline with ammonia and volume is made up to 50ml. After making up the volume the solution is allowed to stand for 5 minutes so that a colour develops which is viewed vertically and compared with the standard solution.

2. Standard Solution: 40ml of water is added to 2ml of standard solution of iron. Then 2ml of 20% w/v citric acid and 2 drops of thioglycolic acid is added to the above solution. The solution is made alkaline with ammonia and volume is made up to 50ml. The resultant solution is allowed to stand for 5 minutes so that a colour develops which is viewed vertically and compared with the test solution.

When the colour of both the solutions is compared, the intensity of the colour of the test solution should be less than that of the standard solution.

Some **essential point**s that should be kept in mind while performing the limit test of iron are as follows:

1. Colour is developed and not turbidity.
2. The solutions should be compared immediately within 5 minutes, else the colour fades away due to oxidation, making the test unreliable.
3. Mercapto acetic acid test is very sensitive.

Q.18. Discuss the principle and reaction involved in the limit test of Arsenic.

Limit Test for Arsenic (I.P. 1996): This test is carried out for controlling the arsenic impurity in inorganic substances.

Principle: The limit test for arsenic (a modification of the **Gutzeit test**) is based on the reaction in which arsenic is converted to arsine (ASH) by undergoing reduction with zinc and hydrochloric acid. The use of stannate hydrochloric acid, i.e., stannous chloride mixed with hydrochloric acid is prescribed in the I.P.

$$H_3AsO_4 \rightarrow H_3AsO_3$$
$$H_3AsO_4 + 6H_2 \rightarrow AsH_3\uparrow 3H_2O$$

When arsine comes in contact with dry paper saturated with mercuric chloride/bromide, it produces a yellow or brown stain.

$$2AsH_3 + HgCl_2 \rightarrow Hg2AsH_2 + HCl$$

The intensity of the color produced is proportional to the amount of In the arsenic present, if the diameter of the paper exposed to arsine is constant. The test solution of the sample is compared with the standard solution with known amount of arsenic. The stains are then compared in natural light (i.e., daylight).

Apparatus: A wide-mouthed flask or bottle of 120ml is fitted with a rubber bung and a glass tube passes through it, having a total length of 200mm, internal diameter of 6.5mm and external diameter of 8mm. At one end to a diameter of 1mm the tube is drawn out and near the constricted part a hole of about 2mm in diameter is blown in the side of the tube. When the cork (stopper) is inserted in the bottle containing 70ml of liquid, the constricted end of the tube is above the surface of the liquid, and the hole in the side is below the bottom of the cork. The upper end of the tube is slightly rounded.

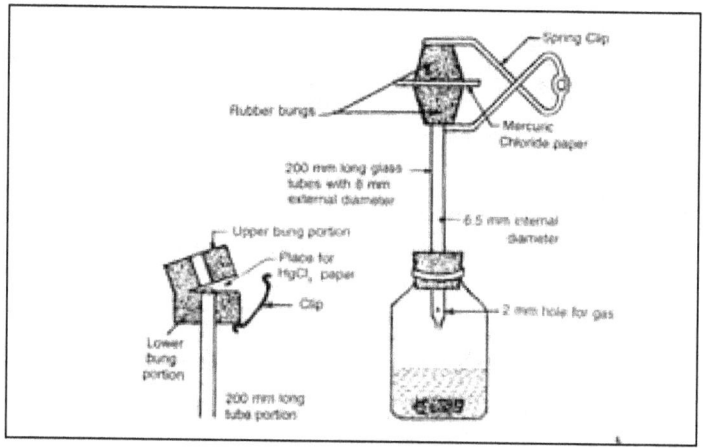

Two rubber cork (about 25mmx25mm), each with a hole of 6.5mm in diameter at the centre, and a tube are fitted with a rubber band or spring clip for holding them tightly together. The two corks may be replaced by any suitable device in order to satisfy the conditions.

During the test, the gas released passes through the side hole; and hole on lower side acts as an exit for water which condenses in the tube.

Procedure: In this limit test, a standard solution and test solution is prepared and the appearance of these two solutions is compared:

1. Test Solution: The test solution is prepared as directed in the monograph and placed in the generator bottle. 5ml of 1M potassium iodide, 5ml of stannous chloride acid solution, and 10gm of zine AST are added to the test solution. A test paper of mercuric chloride is placed in the rubber slit and the bottle is immediately stoppered. The reaction is allowed to continue for 40 minutes at about 40°C.

2. Standard Solution (10ppm as): 0.33gm of arsenic trioxide is dissolved in 5ml of 2M NaOH (sodium hydroxide) solution and volume is made up to 250ml with water. 1ml of this solution is further diluted with distilled water up to 100ml. The stain produced by the test sample is compared with the standard stain. The sample passes the test, if the stain produced by it is less intense than that of the standard.

The standard dilute arsenic solution with 0.132gm of As_2O_3 per 100ml solution is prepared. 1ml of the above solution is diluted with 100ml of water to prepare a dilute arsenic solution (1ml of which would be having 0.00001gm of as).

A stain equivalent to 1ml of the dilute arsenic solution produced by operating on 10gm of the substance would, therefore, show that the proportion of arsenic has been 1ppm ($0.00001g/10=1\times10^{-6}$).

Reagents: Letter 'AST" is used to mark and distinguish all the reagents used in the test. AST signifies that all the reagents should be free from arsenic a should conform to its limit test.

Precautions:

1. The standard stain should be compared immediately as it fades away or standing.
2. Arsenic chloride paper should be stored in a dark place as it undergoes discoloration when exposed to light, thus, making it unfit to be used is the test.
3. The tube should be washed with hydrochloric acid 'AST", then with water, and dried between the consequent tests.

Q.19. Discuss the principle and reaction involved in the limit test of Lead.

Limit Test for Lead (I.P. 1996): This test is carried out for controlling the lead impurity in inorganic substances.

Principle: The limit test for lead relies on the formation of a complex by the reaction between lead and diphenyl thiocarbazone (dithizone). A chloroform solution of dithizone is prepared, which extracts lead from alkaline aqueous S solutions, forming a red-colored lead dithizone complex.

Amount of lead present in the solution influences the intensity of the complex. The colour of lead-dithizone complex in chloroform and in the standard lead solution is compared.

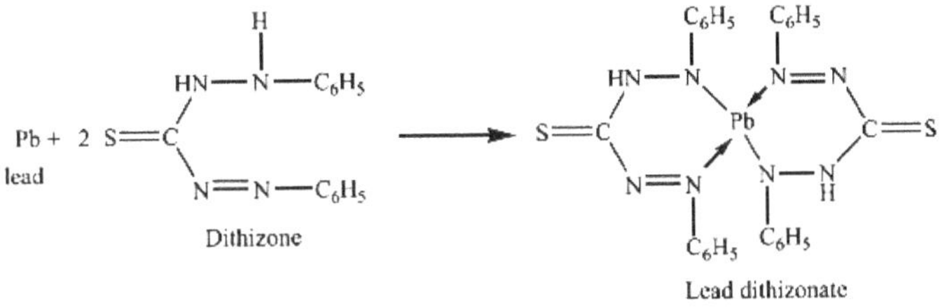

Pb + 2 — lead

Dithizone

Lead dithizonate

In this method, addition of ammonium citrate, potassium cyanide, and hydroxylamine hydrochloride complexes the metallic impurities (especially, iron) which do not interfere with the extraction of lead.

Procedure: In this limit test, a standard solution and test solution is prepared and the appearance of these two solutions is compared:

1. Test Solution: The sample solution is prepared as prescribed in the monograph and taken in a separating funnel. Then 6ml of ammonium citrate (40gm citric acid in 90ml water and ammonia solution) and 2ml of hydroxylamine hydrochloride (20gm in 100ml water) are added. followed by 2 drops of phenol red. Ammonia solution is added to make the resultant solution alkaline. Other metals are complexed by adding 2ml of potassium cyanide solution (10gm potassium cyanide in each 100ml).

About 5ml dithizone solution (30ml dithizone in 1litre of $CHCl_3$) is used to extract the above solution until it becomes green. With 20ml of 1% nitric acid, the combined dithizone extracts are shaken for 30 seconds, converting all the lead dithizone into nitrate.

The remaining chloroform layer is discarded and again extracted with 5ml of dithizone extraction solution in the presence of 94ml of ammonium cyanide and the solution is shaken for 30 seconds.

2. Standard Solution: A standard solution is prepared similarly with a volume of dilute standard lead solution equivalent to the amount of lead permitted in the sample being tested and containing all other reagents in the same quantity as in the test solution.

The colour of the chloroform layer developed in the test sample should not be of deeper shade of violet than that of standard.

Some **essential points** that should be kept in mind while performing the limit test of lead are as follows:

1. In this test, all the reagents and solutions used should be free from lead (designated as PbT).
2. Glassware should be washed properly with warm dilute HNO, and then with water.

Q.20. Discuss the principle and reaction involved in the limit test of Heavy Metals.

Limit Test for Heavy Metals (I.P. 1996): This limit test is carried out for determining the content of metallic impurities coloured by sulphide ion, under specific conditions. The monographs prescribe the limit for heavy metals in terms of amount of lead parts per million of the substance (by weight).

This has been determined by visually comparing the colour produced by the substance with that of a control prepared from a standard lead solution.

Principle: Limit tests for heavy metals are based on the reaction between a solution of a heavy metal and a saturated solution of H_2S in an acidic medium. A reddish/black colour resulted is compared with the standard solution of lead nitrate solution.

$$Pb+ H_2S \rightarrow PbS+H_2$$

Procedure: Following are the methods which are prescribed in monographs and can be used for determining the amount of heavy metals:

1. Method A: This method is suitable for substances producing clear a colorless solution under the prescribed test conditions.

Standard Solution: 2ml of the standard lead solution is pipetted out in 50ml Nessler cylinder and diluted up to 25ml with water. The pH adjusted between 3-4 using dilute acetic acid or dilute ammonia solution. After pH adjustment the solution is diluted up to 35ml with water.

Test Solution: 25ml of test solution is prepared in a 50ml Nessler cylinder and pH is adjusted between 3-4 using dilute acetic acid or dilute ammonia solution. After pH adjustment the solution is diluted a upto 35ml with water.

Procedure: 10ml of freshly prepared hydrogen sulphide solution is added into both the cylinders containing standard and test solution and diluted up to 50ml with water. After dilution the solution is kept aside over a white surface for 5 minutes and viewed downwards. The test solution colour is lighter than the standard solution colour.

2. Method B: This method is suitable for substances not producing clear and colourless solutions under the test conditions prescribed for **method A** or for substances which hinder the precipitation of metals by sulphide ion due to their complex nature.

Standard Solution: 2ml of standard lead solution is pipetted out in a 50ml Nessler cylinder and diluted up to 25ml with water. The pH is adjusted between 3-4 using dilute acetic acid or dilute ammonia solution. After pH adjustment, the solution is diluted up to 35ml with water.

Test Solution: The sample to be tested is weighed in a crucible, wetted with sulphuric acid and burnt by carefully igniting at a low temperature. 2ml of nitric acid and 5 drops of sulphuric acid are added to the burnt mass. The resultant mixture is heated with full care until white fumes stop evolving and then ignited in a muffle furnace at 500-600°C until the carbon is completely burnt off. After cooling. 4ml hydrochloric acid is added to the mixture, covered and digested for 15 minutes on a water-bath. After 15 minutes the mixture is uncovered and evaporated to dryness on a water-bath.

A drop of hydrochloric acid is added to moisten the residue. Then 10ml of hot water is added and the mixture is digested for 2 minutes. The solution is made alkaline by adding ammonia solution drop wise till the solution turns litmus paper blue. The solution is then diluted up to 25ml with water and pH is adjusted between the range of 3-4 by using dilute acetic acid. After adjusting the pH, the solution is filtered (if required). the crucible is rinsed and filtered with 10ml of water. The filtrate and washings are combined in a 50ml Nessler cylinder, diluted up to 35mlwith water and mixed.

Procedure: The procedure is similar to the one employed in **Method A**.

3. Method C: This method is suitable for substances producing clear and colourless solutions with solution of sodium hydroxide.

Standard Solution: 2ml of standard lead solution is pipetted out in a 50ml Nessler cylinder. 5ml of dilute sodium hydroxide solution is added to it and diluted up to 50ml with water.

Test Solution: 25ml of test solution is prepared and placed in a 50ml Nessler cylinder. The quantity prescribed is dissolved in a mixture of 20ml of water and 5ml of dilute sodium hydroxide solution. The resultant solution is diluted up to 50ml with water.

Procedure: 5 drops of sodium sulphide solution are added to each cylinder containing the standard and the test solution. After mixing the cylinders are allowed to stand for 5 minutes over a white surface and viewed downwards. The test solution colour is lighter than that of the standard solution.

Q.21. Discuss the principle and reaction involved in the Modified limit test of Chloride.

Principle: The limit test of chloride is based on the precipitation reaction. The precipitates of chlorides develop on the reaction of soluble chloride with silver nitrate in the presence of dilute nitric acid to form silver chloride, which appears as solid particles (opalescence) in the solution. The intensity of turbidity depends on the number of chlorides present in the test substance.

$$HCl + AgNO_3 \rightarrow AgCl + HNO_3$$

Procedure: With reference to International Pharmacopoeia 6th Edition 2016, the limit test of chloride has been modified in the context of standard solution preparation. Earlier the standard solution of chloride was prepared by dissolving sodium chloride (NaCl, known Cl− impurity) but now it has been modified by using hydrochloric acid (HCl) instead of sodium chloride (NaCl).

Conclusion: If opalescence produced in the sample solution is less than the standard solution, the sample will pass the limit test of chloride and vice versa

Q.22. Discuss the principle and reaction involved in the Modified limit test of Sulphate.

Principle: The principle involved in the limit test for sulphates is the precipitation method. The sulfates are precipitated as barium sulfate by reacting with barium chloride in the presence of hydrochloric acid. The hydrochloric acid used prevents the reaction of other acid radicals with barium chloride as in the presence of hydrochloric acid, only sulfates are precipitated.

$$SO_4^{2-} + BaCl_2 \rightarrow BaSO_4 + 2Cl^-$$

Due to the formation of precipitates, the solution appears turbid and the extent of turbidity depends on the number of sulfates present. If the turbidity produced by the test is less than that of the standard, it means that the sample contains sulfates within prescribed limits.

Reagent Preparations:

1. **Barium Sulphate Reagent:** Dissolve 12g of barium chloride (BaCl2.2H2O) in 1000 ml of water to make 0.05M barium chloride solution. To 15 ml of the prepared solution, add 55 ml water, 20 ml alcohol, 5 ml of 0.0181% w/v potassium sulfate (K2SO4) solution, and makeup the volume up to 100 ml.

2. **Standard Potassium Sulphate Solution:** Accurately weighed 0.1089g of K2SO4 and the volume was made up to 100 ml with water.

Test sample:

1. **Sodium Chloride:** Dissolve 2g of sodium chloride in 20 ml of water.

2. **Sodium bicarbonate:** Dissolve 2g of sodium bicarbonate in little quantity of water.

Procedure: With reference to International Pharmacopoeia 6th Edition 2016, the limit test for sulfate has been modified to a great extent. It has done away the requirement of barium sulfate reagent. However, it still uses alcohol along with barium chloride to produce comparable turbidity.

Conclusion: If the opalescence produced in the standard is more than that of the test, the sample complies with the limit test of sulfate as per I.P. 1996.

UNIT – 2
2.1. Acid, Bases, and Buffers

Q.1. Write different theories of acids and bases.

Acids and Bases: For thousands of years, the sour taste of various foods (like vinegar, lemon juice, tamarind, etc.) had known, but it is only a few hundred years back researchers came to know that the sour taste is due to the acids. The word 'acid' comes from the Latin term *acere* which means 'sour'.

In the 17th century, **Robert Boyle**, an Irish writer and an amateur chemist first labelled substances either as acids or bases, on the basis of the following characteristics:

1. **Acids:** These substances taste sour, are corrosive to metals, change litmus (a dye extracted from lichens) to red, and on mixing with bases become less acidic.
2. **Bases:** These are slippery in nature, change litmus blue, and their basic property decreases on mixing with acid.

Theories: There are three theories, explaining the concept of acids and bases:

1. Arrhenius's theory,
2. Bronsted-Lowry theory, and
3. Lewis theory.

Overview of the Three Theories

Theory	Acid	Base
Arrhenius	H^+ producer	OH^- producer
Bronsted-Lowry	H^+ donor	H^+ acceptor
Lewis	Electron pair acceptor	Electron pair donor

1. Arrhenius Theory:

The most commonly used concept of acids and bases was developed by **Savante Arrhenius** in 1884, termed **Arrhenius Theory**. According to this theory, an **acid** is a substance which dissociates in an aqueous solution and produces hydrogen ions (H^+).

On other hand, a base is a substance which dissociates in aqueous solution to produce hydroxyl ion (OH^-).

For example, HCI is an Arrhenius acid and NaOH is an Arrhenius base

$$HCl_{(aq.)} \rightarrow H^+_{(aq.)} + Cl^-_{(aq.)}$$
$$NaOH_{(aq.)} \rightarrow OH^-_{(aq.)} + Na^+_{(aq.)}$$

Arrhenius's theory was the first scientific theory that had given definitions for acids and bases as well as classified them. It is the simplest theory and is useful in the case of aqueous solutions.

Limitations: Chemical reactions can be studied well by using acid-base theory of Arrhenius but it has some limitations:

1. Acids and bases have been defined only in terms of solution and not as solid substances.

2. This theory failed in elaborating the acidic and basic properties of a substance in non-aqueous solvents, e.g., NH_4NO_3 does not give H^+ ions but acts as an acid in liquid NH_3.

3. This theory also failed to explain the neutralization of acid and base in the absence of solvent.

4. There are many basic substances (few organic substances and NH_3) which do not have OH^- ions but are basic in nature. This fact could not be explained by **Arrhenius** theory.

5. Acidic properties of many salts ($AlCl_3$ in aqueous solution) could not be explained by this theory.

2. Bronsted-Lowry Theory:

J.N. Bronsted and **J.M. Lowry** in 1923 gave a broader concept of acids and bases, independently. According to this theory, an **acid** is any molecule or ion that can donate a proton (H^+) and a **base** is any molecule or ion that can accept a proton.

An acid is a proton donor, while base is a proton acceptor. A **base** qualifying Bronsted-Lowry concept is termed as **Bronsted-Lowry base** or **Bronsted base**, whereas an **acid** qualifying termed as Bronsted-Lowry concept is termed as **Bronsted-Lowry acid** or **Bronsted acid**.

For example, on dissolving dry HCl gas in water, each molecule of HCl produces a hydronium ion by donating a proton to a water molecule.

$$H_2O + HCl \rightarrow H_3O^+ + Cl$$

Therefore, it can be concluded that water which accepts a proton is a **Bronsted base**, whereas HCl gas which donates a proton is a **Bronsted acid**.

Conjugate Acid-Base Pairs: The acid (HA) involved in an acid-base reaction produces a new base (A⁻) by donating its proton (H⁺). This new base is called the **conjugate base** which is related to the original acid. Similarly, after accepting a proton (H⁺) the original base (B⁻) produces a new acid (HB) known as the **conjugate acid**.

The acid (HA) and the conjugate base (A⁻) together constitute a conjugate acid-base pair as they are related to each other by donating and accepting a single proton. The above acid-base reaction shows two pairs of conjugate acid-base, i.e., HA and A⁻ and HB and B⁻.

Advantages: The Bronsted-Lowry theory has many advantages over Arrhenius theory a given below:

1. **Much Wider Scope:** Bronsted-Lowry concept of acids and bases covers wider range of molecules and ions accepting proton (bases) or donating proton (acids). Whereas, Arrhenius concept of acids and bases involves only those substances which release H or OH ions in aqueous solution.

2. **Not Limited to Aqueous Solutions:** Arrhenius concept is limited only to aqueous solutions but Bronsted-Lowry model not only covers aqueous solutions but also gas phase.

For example, ammonium chloride is obtained by the reaction between gaseous ammonia (a Bronsted base) and hydrogen chloride gas (a Bronsted acid).

$$NH3 + HCl \rightarrow NH4^+ + Cl^-$$

In this reaction, a proton donated by HCl is accepted by NH_3. But according to Arrhenius model, this is not considered as an acid-base reaction.

3. **Release of OH not Necessary to Qualify as a Base:** Bronsted base is a substance which accepts a proton, whereas Arrhenius base is a substance which releases OH ions in aqueous solution.

   For example, liquid ammonia (NH_3) is a base but does not releases OH⁻ ions in water. But as per Bronsted-Lowry theory, it is a base as it forms NH_4^+ (an acid) by accepting a proton.

$$NH_3 + H^+ \longleftarrow\!\longrightarrow NH_4^+$$

Limitations: The Bronsted-Lowry Theory has mainly two limitations as given below:

1. Bronsted-Lowry theory of acids and bases is based on transfer of protons. Commonly most of the acids are protonic in nature but some are not.

2. There is no transfer of protons in acid-base chemical reactions, therefore, the reactions occurring in non-protonic solvents cannot be explained by the protonic definitions, **e.g.,** $COCl_2$, SO_2, N_2O_4, etc.

3. Lewis Theory of Acids and Bases:

A more general model of acids and bases was given by **G.N. Lewis** in the early **1930s**. He defined **acid** as an electron-pair acceptor and **base** as an electron-pair donor.

In this theory, the Lewis acid and Lewis base shares an electron pair given by base resulting in the formation of a covalent or coordinate bond between them. This resultant compound bonded with a covalent bond is known as a **complex**. If the Lewis acid is denoted by A and the Lewis base by B, the fundamental equation of the Lewis theory can be represented as:

$$\underset{\textbf{Lewis acid}}{\textbf{A}} \ + \ \underset{\textbf{Lewis base}}{\textbf{:B}} \ \rightarrow \ \underset{\textbf{Complex}}{\textbf{A— B}}$$

According to this concept:

1. Lewis bases are anions or molecules having a lone pair of electrons,
2. Lewis acids are cations or molecules lacking an electron pair

Examples of Lewis Reactions

1. Between H^+ and NH_3: Proton (H^+) can accept an electron pair, thus is a Lewis acid. Ammonia molecule ($:NH_3$) has an electron-pair to donate, thus is a Lewis base. The Lewis reaction occurring between H^+ and NH_3 can be represented as:

$$\underset{\textbf{Lewis acid}}{\textbf{H}^+} \ + \ \underset{\textbf{Lewis base}}{\textbf{NH}_3} \ \longleftrightarrow \ \underset{\textbf{Complex}}{\textbf{NH}_4{}^+}$$

2. **Between H⁺ and OH⁻:** The proton (H^+) is a Lewis acid being an electron-pair acceptor, whereas, OH^- is a Lewis base being an electron-pair donor. The Lewis reaction occurring between H^+ and OH^- can be represented as:

$$H^+ \qquad + \ [O-H]^- \qquad \longleftrightarrow \qquad H-O-H$$

$$\text{Lewis acid} \qquad \text{Lewis base} \qquad\qquad \text{Complex}$$

Advantages:

1. It explains the acidic and basic nature on the basis of or of electrons accompanied by loss/donation of electron pair.
2. It includes the definitions given by both Arrhenius and Bronsted-Lowry.
3. It overcame the disadvantages Bronsted-Lowry theory; CO_2 could now encompass the definition of an acid.

Limitations:

1. Lewis acids and bases cannot be arranged in their order of strength as their strength depends on the reaction type.
2. Due to involvement of electrons in Lewis acids and bases, their reactions are assumed to be very fast but some of the Lewis acid-base reactions are slow.

Q.2. Give Pharmaceutical importance of Acids and Bases.

Acids and Bases: For thousands of years, the sour taste of various foods (like vinegar, lemon juice, tamarind, etc.) had known, but it is only a few hundred years back researchers came to know that the sour taste is due to the acids. The word 'acid' comes from the Latin term *acere* which means 'sour'.

In the 17th century, **Robert Boyle**, an Irish writer and an amateur chemist first labelled substances either as acids or bases, on the basis of the following characteristics:

1. **Acids:** These substances taste sour, are corrosive to metals, change litmus (a dye extracted from lichens) to red, and on mixing with bases become less acidic.
2. **Bases:** These are slippery in nature, change litmus blue, and their basic property decreases on mixing with acid.

Pharmaceutical Importance of Acids and Bases: Acids, bases, and their reactions have an important role in pharmaceutical studies and preparations. A few of their main uses are as follows:

1. Acid-base neutralization reactions are used in the preparation of suitable salts, and in the transformation of salts into their more suitable forms. A specific acid-base system is used to prepare effervescent mixtures.
2. In analytical chemistry, various acids and bases are used during acid- base titrations.
3. Various acids and bases are found in human body and used as therapeutic agents to maintain the pH of GIT, urine, blood and other body fluids

4. Buffers are conjugate pairs of acids or bases. **For example**, buffer base acts as a proton acceptor, and buffer acid acts as a proton donor.

Q.3. What is Buffer Solution? Give its characteristics and types.

Buffers: A solution is said to be a buffer solution, if its pH remains unchanged or shows very slight changes, when a small amount of either an acid (H^+ ions) or a base (OH^- ions) is added. A buffer solution can also be defined as a solution which resists pH changes on addition of small amount of acid or alkali due to its reserved acidity or alkalinity property.

The activity of buffer solution can be explained by an **example** of 1 liter of an aqueous sodium chloride solution. This solution has pH 7 which reduces to 3, when 1ml of 1M HCl solution is added to it and becomes one liter when 1ml of 1M NaOH solution is added to it. Thus, it can be concluded that sodium chloride solution is not a buffer.

In another an aqueous ammonium acetate solution (1 liter) has pH7. On adding the same amount of acid (1ml of 1M HCl) or alkali (1ml of 1M NaOH), the pH does not undergo any change and remains the same, i.e., 7. Thus, ammonium acetate solution resists change in its pH on addition of an acid or a base, and is a buffer solution.

Characteristics of Buffer Solution: Buffer solution possesses a few characteristic features:

1. Since, it has reserve acidity or alkalinity, thus, a definite pH.
2. Even when stored for a long duration, its pH does not change.

3. There is no alteration in its pH on dilution.

4. When small amount of an acid or a base is added, its pH changes slightly.

Types of Buffer Solution: Buffer solutions or buffers resist pH changes or undergo a slight pH change, when small amount of an acid or base is added to it. **Buffer solutions** are of the following **types**:

1. **Acid Buffers:** A weak acid and its salt with a strong base, e.g., $CH_3COOH + CH_3COONa$.

2. **Basic Buffers:** A weak base and its salt with a strong acid, e.g., $NH_4OH + NH_4Cl$

Q.4. Define buffer with buffer capacity?

Buffers: A solution is said to be a buffer solution, if its pH remains unchanged or shows very slight changes, when a small amount of either an acid (H^+ ions) or a base (OH^- ions) is added. A buffer solution can also be defined as a solution which resists pH changes on addition of small amount of acid or alkali due to its reserved acidity or alkalinity property.

Example of 1 liter of an aqueous sodium chloride solution. This solution has pH 7 which reduces to 3, when 1ml of 1M HCl solution is added to it and becomes one liter when 1ml of 1M NaOH solution is added to it. Thus, it can be concluded that sodium chloride solution is not a buffer.

Buffer Capacity: The efficiency of a buffer to resist the changes in pH is called the **buffer capacity (β)**. It can also be defined as the amount of strong acid or base (in gram-equivalents) that must be added to 1litre (one liter) of the buffer solution to change its pH by one unit.

Buffer capacity can be calculated using the following formula:

$$\beta = \frac{\Delta B}{\Delta pH}$$

Where,
ΔB = Gram equivalent of strong acid/base to change the pH of1 liter of buffer solution.
ΔpH= Change in pH by the addition of strong acid/base.

Practically, buffer capacity measures the small changes in pH and is quantitatively expressed as the ratio of acid or base added to the change in pH (**e.g., mEq/pH for x volume**).

Following are the **two factors** which influences the **buffer capacity**:

1. Ratio of the salt to the acid or base. When this ratio is 1:1, i.e.,pH = pKa, buffer capacity is optimal, and
2. Total buffer concentration, **for example**, a 0.5M buffer will require more acid or base for its depletion than a 0.05M buffer.

The relationship between buffer capacity and buffer concentrations is given by **Van Slyke equation**:

$$\beta = 2.3C \frac{K_a[H_3O^+]}{(K_a + [H_3O^+])^2}$$

Where,
C = Total buffer concentration (i.e., the sum of the molar concentrations of acid and salt).

Q.5. Write buffer equation with its significance and limitations.

Buffer Equation (Henderson-Hasselbalch Equation): A weak acid (HA) dissociates as follows:

$$HA = 2.3 \leftrightarrow H^+ + A^-$$

$$\text{and} \quad K_a = \frac{[H^+][A^-]}{[HA]}$$

$$\text{or} \quad [H^+] = K_a \times \frac{[HA]}{[A^-]} \quad ....(1)$$

The weak acid (HA) undergoes slight dissociation. Addition of the salt (Na$^+$ A$^-$) to this weak acid results to common ion effect as it provides a common ion, i.e., A$^-$ion. This property further depresses the dissociation of the weak acid. This results in equality between the equilibrium concentration of the unionized acid A and the initial concentration of the acid. It is also assumed that equality exists between the equilibrium concentration A and the salt's initial concentration (when added) as it dissociates Therefore, **equation (1)** can be written as:

$$[H^+] = K_a \times \frac{[Acid]}{[Salt]} \quad .... (2)$$

Where,
[Acid]= Initial concentration of the added acid
[Salt]= Initial concentration of the salt used

On taking negative logs on both the sides of **equation (2)**:

$$-\log [H^+] = -\log K_a - \log \frac{[Acid]}{[Salt]} \quad ....(3)$$

$$\text{But} \quad -\log [H^+] = pH \quad \text{and} \quad \log K_a = pK_a$$

Therefore, **equation (3)** becomes:

$$pH = pK_a - \log \frac{[Acid]}{[Salt]} = pK_a + \log \frac{[Acid]}{[Salt]}$$

Hence $\quad pH = pK_a + \log \dfrac{[Acid]}{[Salt]}$ .... (4)

The relationship depicted in **equation (4)** is the **Henderson-Hasselbalch Equation** or **Henderson Equation** for an **acidic buffer**.

Similarly, the **Henderson-Hasselbalch equation for a basic buffer** can be represented as:

$$pOH = pK_b + \log \frac{[Acid]}{[Salt]}$$ ....(5)

Significance: Henderson-Hasselbalch equation has the following significant features:

1. Initial concentrations of the weak acid and the salt (if the value of Ka is given) can be used to determine the pH of a buffer solution.

2. The pH of a buffer solution containing equal concentrations of the acid or base and salt can be used to determine the dissociation constant of a weak acid or a weak base.

$$pH = pKc + \log \frac{[Salt]}{[Acid]}$$

$$\text{since } [Salt] = [Acid], \log \frac{[Salt]}{[Acid]} = \log 1 = 0$$

$$\therefore pKc = pH$$

3. The pKa value of weak acid can be determined from the pH obtained

4. By making suitable adjustments in the concentrations of the salt and acid added, a buffer solution of desired pH can be obtained.

Limitations: Among the various approximations implied on Henderson-Hasselbalch equation, the most significant is to assume that at equilibrium the concentration of acid and its conjugate base will be equal to that of the formal concentration. Thus, on neglecting the acid dissociation and the base hydrolysis, the dissociation of water also gets neglected.

These approximations however fail on using strong acids or bases (pK_a more than a couple units away from 7), dilute or very concentrated solutions (less than 1mM or greater than 1M), or heavily skewed acid/base ratios (more than 100 to 1).

Q.6. Write a note on buffer in pharmaceutical system with two examples.

Buffers in Pharmaceutical Systems: Pharmaceutical buffers are used to preserve pH limits in pharmaceutical preparations. In some specific pharmaceutical preparations, in order to maintain the chemical stability and solubility of their ingredients, the pH is needed to be preserved.

Properties: A buffer to be used in the pharmaceutical preparations should possess the following properties:

1. It should remain unaffected in the presence of active ingredients, and other additives.
2. It should not undergo any chemical reactions, like redox reactions, hydrolysis reactions, etc.
3. It should not have any effect on the solubility of other ingredients
4. It should be safe and should not have any influence on pharmacological actions of active ingredients.

Examples: Phosphate Buffer: It is a physiologically compatible buffer solution with pK_a value of the dihydrogen phosphate anion 7.2. This value is almost equal to lacrimal fluid and physiological fluids, thus making it an efficient buffer system.

Disadvantages:

1. Many cations (like Ag. Al. Zn) are insoluble in this buffer. Therefore, it cannot be used in the preparation of collyrium and gargles of zinc salts. If taken internally, it can precipitate calcium. iron and magnesium in the intestine.
2. Phosphate buffer facilitates mold growth at room temperature. By storing the buffer in a refrigerator, the mold growth can be prevented for a reasonable time period. It is generally added with 0.002% benzalkonium chloride, or benzethonium chloride.
3. Sorenson phosphate buffer is a modified phosphate buffer. It is prepared by adding sodium chloride which makes it isotonic with the physiological fluid.

2. Borate Buffer:
It is generally used with those pharmaceutical preparations in which metals get precipitated in case of phosphate buffers.

Disadvantages:

1. Due to toxic nature, boric acid and borate are not used in the preparation of injectable and other internal formulations.
2. This system is inefficient at physiological pH since pK_a value of boric acid is 9.2. Borates have weak bacteriostatic properties, but they facilitate mold growth at room temperature.

Borate buffer systems presently used in pharmaceutical preparations are:

1. Feldman's buffer (pH 7-8.2),
2. Atkins and Pantin buffer (pH 7.6-11), and
3. Gifford's buffer (pH 6-7.8)

Revised Feldman Buffer Mixtures:

Acid buffer solution	Boric acid, N.F. Sodium	12.4gm
	Chloride, U.S.P. Purified	2.9gm
	Water, q.s.	1000ml
Alkaline buffer	Sodium Borate, U.S.P.	19.07gm
	Purified Water, q.s.	1000ml

Q.7. Write a note on Preparation and Stability of Buffer Solution.

Preparation of Buffer Solution: Buffer solutions can be prepared by the following methods:

1. By mixing a weak acid and its salt with a strong base,

   Examples:

   a) $CH_3COOH + CH_3COONa$

   b) Boric acid + Borax

   c) Phthalic acid + Potassium acid phthalate

2. By mixing a weak base and its salt with a strong acid,

   Examples:

   a) $NH_4OH + NH_4Cl$

   b) Glycine + Glycine hydrochloride

3. From an ampholyte solution or amphoteric electrolytes which show both acidic and basic property,

   Examples: Proteins and amino acids.

4. By mixing an acid salt and a normal salt of a polybasic acid,

   Examples: $Na_2HPO_4 + Na_3PO_4$

5. By mixing a salt of weak acid and a weak base,

   Examples: CH_3COONH_4

Stability: Generally, shelf-life of an unopened commercial technical buffer is 2years, and for an opened commercial buffer is 3-6 months. However, this is not applicable to alkaline buffers (pH buffer 10 or higher). It is because changes in pH of alkaline solutions can be observed markedly when they come into contact with CO_2 in the air.

Therefore, it is advisable to:

1. Check the expiration date of the pH buffer solution. The label of the package or at the concerned certificate of analysis must be checked properly. The expired buffer should be prohibited.
2. Keep the buffer solutions in closed plastic containers or inside stoppered flasks/bottles.
3. Store the buffer solution at room temperature (15-30°C) or refrigerate at2-8°C.
4. Label (with manufacturing and expiration date) the buffer solution after its preparation.

The bottles containing alkaline buffers should be stored in the refrigerator but anything may produce carbon dioxide must not be there. The evaporation of the water in the buffer is slower at lower temperatures than at higher temperatures. Thus, the concentration of the buffer solution remains constant for a longer time period.

It is advisable to maintain the buffer solution at room temperature prior to use. The buffer solution must not be kept near window or a heat source.

Q.8. Write a short note on Buffered Isotonic Solutions with suitable example.

Buffered Isotonic Solutions: The pH of pharmaceutical solutions that are meant to be applied on the delicate membranes of the body must be adjusted nearly to the same osmotic pressure as that of the body fluids. After coming in contact with the body tissue, the isotonic solutions do not cause swelling or tissue contraction. These buffered isotonic solutions should not produce any discomfort when instilled in nasal passage, eye, blood, or other body tissues.

The isotonic property of solutions that are meant to be applied to delicate membranes can be explained by mixing a minute quantity of blood in aqueous NaCl solution of variable tonicity.

For example, if blood cells retain their normal size on mixing with a solution containing 0.9gm of NaCl per 100ml, the solution has the same salt concentration. Therefore, they have same osmotic pressure as the RBCs and are recognized to be isotonic with the blood.

If the RBCs are mixed in a solution of 2.0% NaCl, the water content of cells passes through the cell membrane in order to dilute the surrounding salt solution until the salt concentrations on both sides of the cell membrane becomes equal.

Thus, outward movement of water causes shrinking of cells and make them wrinkled or crescent-shaped. Such salt solutions are recognized as hypertonic solutions with respect to the blood cell contents.

If RBCs are suspended in a 0.2% NaCl solution or with distilled water, the water enters into the blood cell and makes them swell and burst to liberate hemoglobin. This phenomenon is termed as **hemolysis**. The weak salt solution or water is recognized as a **hypotonic solution** with respect to the blood.

Q.9. What is tonicity? Give methods for Measurement of Tonicity.

Tonicity: Tonicity is defined as the concentration of only solutes that are unable to cross the membrane because an osmotic pressure is exerted by the on that membrane.

Measurement of Tonicity:

1. **Haemolytic Method:** This method is based on effects of various solutions of drug on the appearance of RBCs suspended in the solutions. A quantitative method based on the principle of haemolysis was developed by **Hunter**. This method was based on the fact that the oxyhaemoglobin liberated from the hypotonic solution is directly proportional to the number of cells haemolysed. The van't Hoff factor '**i**'is obtained and is compared with the values obtained from cryoscopic data, osmotic coefficient, and activity coefficient.

2. **Measurement of the Slight Temperature Differences:** This method is based on the measurement of slight temperature differences which results from the variations between the vapour pressures of thermally insulated samples present in constant humidity chambers.

   For example, -0.52°C is the freezing point of both human blood and lacrimal fluid. This temperature corresponds to the freezing point of a0.90% NaCl solution, which is therefore considered to be isotonic with both blood and lacrimal fluid.

3. **Calculating Tonicity Using L_{iso} Values:** The freezing point depressions for solutions of electrolytes of both the weak and strong types are always greater than those measured from the

equation $\Delta T_f = K_f C$ Therefore, a new factor, $L = iK_f$ is introduced to overcome this difficulty and the equation becomes:

$$\Delta T_f = LC \ldots\ldots\ldots\ldots\ldots\ldots\ (1)$$

Value of L can be calculated by lowering the freezing point of solution of compound of given ionic type with concentration 'C' prime that is isotonic with the body fluids is used to obtain the L value. This specific value of L is written as L_{iso}.

In case a solution of a 0.90% (0.154M) sodium chloride has a freezing point depression of 0.52°C and is isotonic with body fluids then its L iso value will be 3.4:

$$L_{iso} = \frac{\Delta T_f}{C} \ldots\ldots\ldots\ldots\ldots\ldots\ldots\ldots\ (2)$$

We have:

$$L_{iso} = \frac{0.52°C}{0.154} = 3.4$$

Irrespective of their chemical nature, and if not too concentrated, the inter-ionic attractions in solutions are usually same for all univalent electrolytes. Such compounds of this class are known to exhibit the same L_{iso} value (3.4). Because of this similarity among compounds of a given ionic type, the L_{iso} value for dilute solutions of non-electrolytes is almost equal to K_f.

Q.10. Give Methods of Adjusting Isotonicity with suitable examples.

Calculations and Methods of Adjusting Isotonicity: There are usually two methods for adjusting tonicity that can be sub-divided into the following two classes, i.e., Class I and Class II:

1. **Class I Method:** This method is used in order to make the drug solution isotonic with the body fluids. This method utilizes addition of sodium chloride or some other substances to the drug solution to lower the freezing point of the solution to -0.52°C. This method is further categorized as the:

   a) **Cryoscopic method,**

   b) **Sodium chloride equivalent method:**

a) **Cryoscopic Method:** The information related to colligative properties of solutions is important in the preparation of isotonic solutions. Osmotic pressure, elevation in boiling point, depression in freezing point, and lowering of vapour pressure are few important colligative properties. Depression in freezing point is a practical colligative property and is widely used for adjusting tonicity. The freezing point of both the human blood and lacrimal fluids is − 0.52°C. This temperature is equivalent to freezing point of 0.90% (w/v) sodium chloride solution.

The 0.90% (w/v) sodium chloride solution is considered isotonic with blood and lacrimal fluids. For 1% (w/v) sodium chloride solution, depression in freezing point($\Delta T_f^{1\%}$) will be 0.58°C. This method involves the addition of a tonicity adjuster (like sodium chloride) to drug solution to lower the final freezing point of blood or serum (0.52°C).

Example: Find out the weight of NaCl required to prepare 100ml of a 1% solution of apomorphine hydrochloride isotonic with blood.

Solution: Lowering in freezing point of a 1% solution of apomorphine hydrochloride is 0.08°C.

By adding necessary amount of NaCl, the given solution can be made isotonic. Since NaCl has a freezing point lowering of 0.52°C, the amount of additional lowering required to make solutions isotonic is 0.52 – 0.08 = 0.44°C.

$$\Delta T_f^{1\%} \text{for NaCl is } 0.58°C.$$

Let the amount of NaCl in the final solution required to produce a freezing point depression of 0.52 be x.

By method of ratio and proportions:

$$\frac{1\%}{x} = \frac{0.58}{0.44}$$

$$x = 0.76\%$$

Thus, the final amounts of ingredients to be added to make isotonic solution are:

Apomorphine hydrochloride = 1gm

Sodium chloride = 0.76gm

Water, to make 100ml

b) **Sodium Chloride Equivalent Method:** This method involves calculation of either the sodium chloride equivalent or tonicity equivalent of a drug, i.e., the E-value. It is usually the quantity of sodium chloride whose osmotic effect is equivalent to 1g of the drug.

Derivation of E-Value

Different factors like the number of particles, dissociation and association of particles are known to affect the freezing point depression (colligative property) of a solution.

Therefore, the equation:

$$\Delta T_f = K_f C \dots\dots\dots\dots (1)$$

can be replaced with:

$$\Delta T_f = L_{iso} C \dots\dots\dots\dots (2)$$

Where,

$$\Delta T_f = \text{Depression in freezing point}$$

$$K_f = \text{Freezing point depression constant}$$

$c = $ Concentration

L_{iso} is a factor that is equal to iK_f

Where, i is the vant's Hoff factor

$$L_{iso} = \frac{\Delta T_f}{c} \dots\dots\dots\dots (3)$$

The L_{iso} value for each class of electrolyte at a concentration that is isotonic with body fluids is the same because of the similarity of such compounds and similar interionic interactions.

$$\text{Molarity} = \text{mol}/_L = \frac{\text{Weight (g)}}{\text{Molecular weight} \left(\frac{g}{mol}\right) \text{x Volume (mL)}} \times 1000$$

$$or \quad c = \frac{w}{MW} \times \frac{1000}{v}$$

Where,

w = Weight of solute (g)

MW = Molecular weight of solute (g/mol).

v = Volume of solution (mL)

On substituting in equation (2):

$$\Delta T_f = L_{iso} = \frac{w}{MW} \times \frac{1000}{v} \dots\dots\dots\dots (4)$$

Since, E-value is the amount of NaCl that has the same osmotic effect (i.e., equivalent to) as 1gm of the drug. Therefore,

$$C = \frac{1g}{MW}$$

On substituting in equation (2):

$$\Delta T_f = L_{iso} = \frac{1g}{MW} \dots\dots\dots\dots\dots (5)$$

Example: Find out amount of NaCl equivalent of papaverine hydrochloride, which is a 2-ion electrolyte, dissociating 80% in a given solution (molecular weight of papaverine hydrochloride =376g/mol).

Solution: L_{iso} of papaverine HCl = 2.0

$$E = \frac{17 \times 2.0}{376} = 0.090$$

2. **Class II Method:** This method involves addition of sufficient of water for preparation of an isotonic solution. The final volume of the preparation is made up with an isotonic or a buffered isotonic dilution.

This method is further categorized as

a) **White-Vincent method**

b) Sprowls method:

a) White-Vincent Method: In the class II methods of adjusting tonicity, adequate quantity of water is added to the drugs in order to prepare an isotonic solution. Subsequently the final volume of solution is made up by adding an isotonic or isotonic-buffered diluting vehicle. **White and Vincent** are known to develop certain basic method for performing such calculations. The equation is derived as given below:

For example, In order to prepare 30mL of 1% (w/v) solution of procaine hydrochloride which is isotonic with body fluid (0.3g), weight of the drug (w) is multiplied by the sodium chloride equivalent E.

It is the quantity of NaCl which is osmotically equivalent to 0.3g of procaine hydrochloride:

$$= \textbf{Weight of drug (gm)} \times \textbf{E of drug}................(7)$$
$$= 0.03$$
$$\times 0.21$$
$$= 0.063gm$$

In order to prepare an isotonic solution, approximately 0.9gm of sodium chloride is dissolved in 100mL of water. The volume (V) required for preparing isotonic solution by dissolving 0.063gm of sodium chloride (equivalent to 0.3gm of procaine hydrochloride) is obtained from the following proportion:

$$\frac{0.9g}{100mL} = \frac{0.063g}{V} \quad .... (7)$$

$$V = 0.036 \times {100}/{0.9}$$

$$= 7.0\text{mL}$$

Thus, equation (7) can be written as:

$$V = w \times E \times 111.1 \ldots \ldots \ldots \ldots (8)$$

Here,

V = Volume of isotonic solution (in mL) that is prepared by mixing the drug with water.

w = Weight of the drug (in grams).

B = Sodium chloride equivalent of the drug.

The volume of isotonic solution (ml) is represented by the constant, 111.1, which is obtained by dissolving 1gm of sodium chloride in water.

Equation (8) is used to solve this problem within a single step:

$$V = 0.3 \times 0.21 \times 111.1$$

$$V = 7.0\text{mL}$$

An adequate quantity of isotonic sodium chloride solution or any other isotonic solution is taken and mixed with an isotonic buffered diluted solution to make the final volume up to 30ml. The isotonicity values of the solution and buffered diluting solutions are similar to that of 0.9% NaCl. If more than one ingredient are known to present in an isotonic preparation then the volumes of isotonic solution, isotonic preparation and the volumes of isotonic solution obtained by each drug with water are additive.

Example: Make the following preparation solution isotonic with respect to an ideal membrane.

Phenacaine hydrochloride = 0.06g

Boric acid = 0.30g 100.0mL

Sterilized distilled water q.s. = 100mL

(E for boric acid = 0.50, E for phenacaine hydrochloride = 0.20)

Solution:

$$V = [(0.06 \times 0.20) + (0.3 \times 0.50)] \times 111.1$$
$$V = 18ml$$

Initially the drugs are added in water to make 18ml of an isotonic solution. The resultant solution is further added with an isotonic dilute solution to make the final volume up to 100 ml.

b) **Sprowls Method:** Sprowls further simplifies the method given by **White and Vincent**. According to **Sprowls** the **equation (8)** given by **White and Vincent** can be utilised to illustrate different values of V, while the weight of the drug (w) is kept constant. **Sprowls** selected 0.3gm of drug to prepare one fluid ounce of a 1% solution. Approximately 0.3gm of a drug is mixed with adequate quantity of water to obtain volume (V) of isotonic solution. This solution can be used in the formulation of ophthalmic and parenteral solutions. The required volume of the isotonic solution can be obtained by adding suitable isotonic or isotonic buffered diluting solutions.

Q.11. Find out amount of NaCl should be added to the following formulation to make it isotonic? (molecular weight of pilocarpine nitrate =101g, L_{iso} of pilocarpine nitrate = 0.23g). Pilocarpine nitrate is 0.3g, Sodium chloride q.s., Purified water q.s. is 100mL

Solution: Amount of sodium chloride represented by

pilocarpine nitrate = L_{iso} × **weight of drug (g)**
$$= 0.23 \times 0.3 = 0.069g$$
Amount of NaCl to make 30mL isotonic NaCl solution
$$= 30 \times 0.009$$
$$= 0.270g$$
Amount of NaCl to be used = **0.270 − 0.069**

Q.12. Find out the weight of NaCl required to prepare 100ml of a 1% solution of apomorphine hydrochloride isotonic with blood.

Solution: Lowering in freezing point of a 1% solution of apomorphine hydrochloride is 0.08°C.

By adding necessary amount of NaCl, the given solution can be made isotonic. Since NaCl has a freezing point lowering of 0.52°C, the amount of additional lowering required to make solutions isotonic is 0.52 – 0.08 = 0.44°C.

$$\Delta T_f^{1\%} \text{ for NaCl is } 0.58°C.$$

Let the amount of NaCl in the final solution required to produce a freezing point depression of 0.52 be x.

By method of ratio and proportions:

$$\frac{1\%}{x} = \frac{0.58}{0.44}$$

$$x = 0.76\%$$

Thus, the final amounts of ingredients to be added to make isotonic solution are:

Apomorphine hydrochloride = 1gm

Sodium chloride = 0.76gm

Water, to make 100ml

Q.13. What is Pharmaceutical Buffer? Give Pharmaceutical Importance of Buffers.

Pharmaceutical Buffer: Pharmaceutical buffers are used to preserve pH limits in pharmaceutical preparations. In some specific pharmaceutical preparations, in order to maintain the chemical stability and solubility of their ingredients, the pH is needed to be preserved.

Pharmaceutical Importance of Buffers: In pharmaceutical preparations, buffer solutions play an important role by ensuring stable pH conditions for therapeutically active compounds:

1. **Solubility:** A controlled pH medium is helpful in controlling the solubility of compounds. **For example**, in acidic medium, solubility of different compounds (inorganic salts of Fe^{+3}, phosphates, borates) is increased; but these inorganic salts precipitate in alkaline media.

Likewise, there are many organic compounds which are insoluble in acidic medium but are soluble in alkaline pH, **For example**, alkaloids and amines are soluble in acidic solutions and insoluble in solution of basic pH.

2. **Colour:** The pH of a solution is known to affect the colour of natural dyes, fluid extract and other synthetic drugs. This of colour changing at different pH values is used in identification of various compounds. **For example,** various indicators (**e.g.,** phenolphthalein, phenol sulphonaphthalein) are used on the basis of changes in colour according to the pH.

3. **Stability of Certain Compounds to Redox Conditions:** Many chemical compounds are stable at specific pH range and any variation in pH range may result to processes like auto-oxidation, disproportions, etc. **For example,** ascorbic acid and penicillin are unstable at alkaline pH. In order to prevent the separation of sulphur, sodium thiosulphate and sodium polysulphide preparations are stored at alkaline environment. The formation of coloured nitrogen oxides is responsible for brown colour of nitrites in an acidic media.

4. **Patient Comfort:** Irritation and other severe allergic reactions may occur if the pH of injectable and preparations meant for internal or external use varies largely from the concerned tissue pH. Thus, the existence of strong acidic or alkaline pH may cause tissue damage.

5. **Optimum pH Conditions:** The therapeutic activities of medicinal compounds are more prevalent at specific pH conditions, **e.g.,**

   i. Sodium dihydrogen phosphate is used to buffer methenamine solution.

   ii. Lower pH of sodium hypochlorite usually improves the germicidal efficiency of the preparation.

6. **Study and Research Purpose:** Standard buffers of known pH are used regularly in the analytical laboratory. Standard buffers are required to calibrate pH meter and prepare indicator colour standards.

UNIT – 2

2.2. <u>MAJOR EXTRACELLULAR AND INTRACELLULAR ELECTROLYTES</u>

Q.1. Write a note on Major Extra & Intracellular Electrolytes.

Major Extra & Intracellular Electrolytes: About 56% of the adult human body is fluid. Although most of this fluid is inside the cells and is called intracellular fluid, about one third is in the space outside the cells and is called extracellular fluid. The extracellular fluid is in constant motion throughout the body.

The extracellular fluid has ions and nutrients needed by the cells for the maintenance of life. Therefore, all the cells essentially live in the same environment, i.e., the extracellular fluid. This is the reason that extracellular fluid is called internal environment of the body.

Around 60-70% of the volume of body is water. The fluids in the body are solutions of organic and inorganic solutes which undergo distribution in the following major fluid compartments:

1. Interstitial fluid,

2. Vascular fluid or plasma fluid, and

3. intracellular fluid.

All the body fluids intracellular, extracellular (interstitial, plasma or vascular) contain electrolytes. The electrolyte concentration varies in these fluids, it is 45-50% of body weight in intercellular fluid, interstitial fluid makes 12-15% and plasma makes 4-5% of body weight.

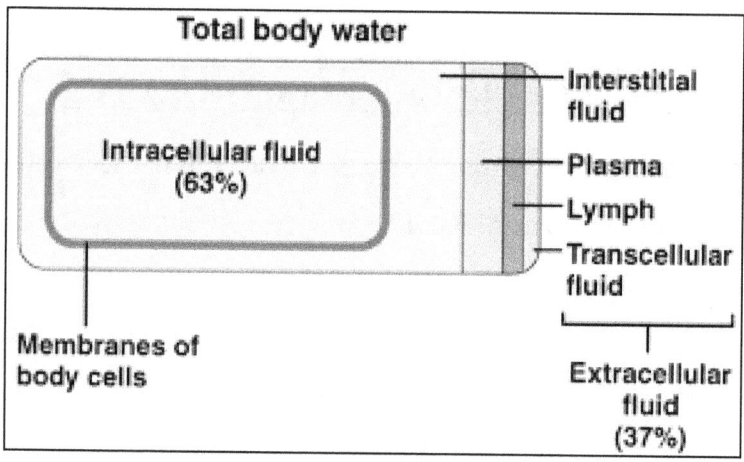

About 40% of intracellular fluid (around 4 liters) is in dense connective tissue, i.e., bone and cartilage and does not take part in quick exchange of electrolytes with the remaining body. The rest of the interstitial fluid (around 6.6 liters) and plasma (around 3.5 liters) comprises the active part of the extracellular fluids.

The extracellular fluid contains large amount of ions (**e.g.,** Na^+, K^+, Cl^-, HCO_3^-, etc.) along with nutrients and other substances for the cell (oxygen, glucose, fatty acids, amino acids, etc.). The intracellular fluid contains large amounts of potassium, magnesium, and phosphate ions.

Q.2. What are electrolytes? Give brief classification of electrolytes.

Electrolytes: Any substance that contains free ions with the property of electrical conductance is known as an **electrolyte**. Electrolytes are also known as **ionic solutions** as they have ions in solution. Electrolytes may exist in both solid and molten electrolyte state.

Electrolytes may be solutions of acids, bases or salts. Some gases under low pressure or high temperature conditions may also act as electrolytes. Dissolution of some synthetic (**e.g.,** polystyrene sulfonate) and biological polymers (**e.g.,** DNA, polypeptides) also result into electrolyte solutions, known as **polyelectrolytes**. These polyelectrolytes possess moieties with multiple charges.

Electrolyte formation can also take place by the process of solvation in which a salt is placed in a solvent (water) and its individual components undergo dissociation, because of the solute and solvent molecules interacting thermodynamically. **For example**, on placing NaCl (table salt) in water, the following reaction occurs:

$$NaCl_{(s)} \rightarrow Na^+ + Cl^-$$

An electrolyte is simply a material that undergoes dissolution in water to form a solution conducting electric current. It is noticeable that the molten salts can also act as electrolytes. **For example**, NaCl in molten allows electrical conductance.

In a solution, an electrolyte is considered to be concentrated if the ions concentration is high; and diluted if the ions concentration is low. An electrolyte is considered to be of high strength, i.e., **strong**, if high amount of solute undergoes dissociation, and of low strength, i.e., **weak**, if most of the solute does not undergo dissociation. The electrolytic properties of electrolyte solutions are used to extract the constituent compounds and elements present in the solution.

Classification of Electrolytes: Electrolytes are substances that dissociate into ions on dissolving in water and conduct electricity. In terms of medicine, it can be defined as dissolved mineral ions, like potassium, chloride, sodium, etc.

Two forces help in the movement of fluids between the compartments:

1. Fluid's hydrostatic pressure, and
2. Substance's osmotic pressure.

Electrolytes are present in the following fluid compartment:

1. Intracellular compartment,
2. Extracellular compartment, and
3. Transcellular compartment.

1. Intracellular Compartment: Intracellular fluid is present within the cell membrane, i.e., in the cell or intracellular compartment. It constitutes 63% of the total body water. General composition of intracellular fluid is:

O_2, more K^+, PO_4^{3-}, Mg^{++}, SO_4^{2-}, less Na^+, Cl^-

Concentration of Important Ions in Intracellular Compartment

Ions	Concentration
K^+	159mM
Na^+	10mM
Cl^-	3mM

Major Intracellular Solutes

1. Proteins (12%),
2. Organic phosphates (18%), and
3. Inorganic ions (64%).

Thus, osmolarity of intracellular compartment is mainly due to the presence of electrolytes.

2. Extracellular Compartment: Extracellular fluid is present outside the cells, i.e., in the extracellular compartment. Extracellular fluid constitutes 37% of the total body water. Blood plasma, interstitial/tissue fluid, and lymph are the examples of fluids present in this compartment. The lymphatic vessels open due to the accumulation of interstitial fluid. This fluid becomes lymph on entering to the open lymphatic vessels and again becomes plasma on returning to the bloodstream.

At equilibrium, an osmotic pressure is present between the intracellular and extracellular compartments. Whenever a change occurs in the osmotic in any of these compartments, fluid exchange takes place between the two. Thus, osmotic pressure provides required pressure for the exchange pressure of fluid between the two compartments.

For example, when sodium (present in high concentration in extracellular fluid) enters the cell, the osmotic pressure within the cell increases. The entry of sodium within the cell is accompanied by water to re-establish equilibrium and balanced osmotic pressure. But, entry of water within the cell causes its swelling. On the other hand, exit of sodium from the cell is also accompanied by water, thus, causing the cell to shrink. General composition of extracellular fluid is:

More Na^+, Cl^-, HCO_3^-, less K^+, Ca^{++}, Mg^{++}, PO_4^{3-}, SO_4^{2-}

Concentration of Important Ions in Extracellular Compartment

Ions	Concentration
K^+	3.5-5.0mM
Na^+	135-145mM
Cl^-	100-111mM

3. Transcellular Compartment: A single epithelial layer separates the extracellular compartment's sub- division, known as transcellular compartment. The **aqueous and vitreous humour of the eye, synovial fluid of the joints, cerebrospinal fluid of the CNS, glandular secretions** and **serous fluid** within the body cavities **(peritoneal and pleural cavities)** are present in this compartment. The transcellular fluids are returned back to the bloodstream after deriving from the plasma.

Q.3. Discuss Physiological Importance of Electrolytes.

Physiological Importance of Electrolytes: Some of the physiological or biological ions are hydrogen phosphate (HPO_4^{2-}), potassium (K^+), chloride (Cl^-), sodium (Na^+) hydrogen carbonate (HCO_3^-), magnesium (Mg^{2+}) and calcium (Ca^{2+}) The ionic nature of the substance is represented by the electric charge symbols of minus (-) and plus (+).

For sustaining life, a continuous balance between extracellular and intracellular environment is necessary. It is essential to maintain electrolyte's precise osmotic gradients in order to maintain a balance between intracellular and extracellular environment. Osmotic gradient regulates the body's hydration, blood pH and also functions of muscles and nerves. In living organisms there are various mechanisms that keep the different electrolyte's concentration under proper and rigid control.

Electrolytes are required in almost every metabolic process of the body, **for example,**

1. Regulation of blood oxygen and pH level, i.e., acidity.
2. Controlling the fluid distribution and water balance in the body.
3. Maintaining an electrical gradient across the cell membranes, crucial for nerve transmission and muscle contraction.
4. Allowing the movement of nutrients within the cells and the waste products out of the cells.

Electrolyte activity between the intracellular fluid and extracellular fluid (interstitial fluid) activates the electrical tissues, i.e., **neurons** and **muscles**. Ion channels are the specialized proteins embedded in the plasma membrane and regulate the movement of electrolytes through the cell membranes. For example, presence of potassium (K^+) sodium (Na^+), and calcium (Ca^+) assists muscle contraction. Absence of sufficient levels of these electrolytes results in muscle twitching and muscle weakness.

Body maintains electrolyte balance by ingesting substances having electrolytes, either orally or intravenously (in emergency cases). Excess amount of electrolytes are flushed out by the kidneys. Human hormones, **e.g.,** aldosterone, antidiuretic hormone and parathyroid hormone, participate in regulation and maintenance of electrolyte homeostasis. Some serious neurological and cardiac complications may result due to over-hydration and dehydration. These complications lead to medical emergency, if not treated immediately.

Q.4. Discuss various functions of Major Physiological Ions.

Major Physiological Ions: Body fluids are found in the form of solutions of organic and inorganic solutes. To maintain homeostasis, all the tissues and cells of body continuously try to maintain the concentration of various components.

An ionic balance exists in the solution of each compartment of the body. Therefore, the extracellular fluid (plasma and interstitial fluids) have sodium and chloride ions, whereas, the intracellular fluid has magnesium, phosphate (as phosphate esters, HPO_4^{2-} and $H_2PO_4^{2-}$) and potassium ions.

Functions of Major Physiological Ions: Following are the **major physiological ions**:

1. Chloride,
2. Phosphate,
3. Bicarbonate,
4. Sodium,
5. Potassium,
6. Calcium, and
7. Magnesium

1. Chloride: In both vascular and interstitial fluid compartments, the **major extracellular anion is chloride (Cl⁻)**. Chloride ions involve in maintenance of osmotic pressure, proper hydration, and normal cation-anion balance.

Main source of chloride is food as it undergoes complete absorption from the intestinal tract. Glomerular filtration helps in the removal of excess chloride from the body, which further undergoes reabsorption in the kidney tubules.

Daily Requirement: Daily requirement of chloride for an adult is about 2.3gm/day.

Dietary Sources: Sea salt or table salt has chloride ions in the form of sodium chloride. Some of the foods having chloride in high amount are rye, lettuce, seaweed, olives, celery, tomatoes, and many vegetables.

In most of the food products, chloride is found in combination with potassium, which is also the main ingredient of salt substitutes.

Functions:

1. The normal cation-anion balance in the compartments with interstitial and vascular fluids is maintained by the chloride ions.
2. The osmotic balance between different fluids of the body is maintained by the chloride ions, along with the sodium ions.
3. Osmotic pressure and proper hydration are also maintained by the chloride ions.
4. The charge balance of the body fluids (extracellular as well as intracellular) is maintained by the chloride ions as they can passthrough all the membranes.
5. Chloride ions are required for the production of HCl in stomach. Here, the Cl⁻ ions passively follow the H⁺ ions (secreted in gastric mucosa by the active transport process) for maintaining electro-neutrality.

2. Phosphate: The **principal intracellular anion** is the phosphate (HPO_4^{2-}), which is present in teeth and bones and also is a crucial buffering system related to calcium, fats and carbohydrates utilization. It exists in concentration of about 80% in divalent HPO_4^{2-} ions form and about 20% in monovalent $H_2PO_4^-$ ions

The physiological processes, such as formation of buffer systems influencing the acid-base balance, lipids and carbohydrates metabolism, energy storage and transfer, and hydrogen ions" renal excretion, demand the involvement of phosphate ions.

Daily Requirement: Daily requirement of phosphate in a normal adult is about 700mg/day.

Dietary Sources: Phosphate can be obtained from protein rich food, like milk and meat.

Functions:

1. Phosphates have mild laxative properties.
2. For proper development of teeth and bones, and proper metabolism of calcium, phosphate ions are essential
3. After phosphorylation, many enzymes work as the coenzymes.
4. Phosphorylation helps in the metabolism of glucose and another hexose.
5. Urine pH is lowered by phosphates, thus given along with certain urinary antimicrobial agents, which depend on acidity of urine.
6. Treatment of hypophosphatemia is done by the phosphates.

3. Bicarbonate: The **second most prevalent extracellular anion** is the **bicarbonate (HPO_3^-).** It is utilized as the most important buffer system of the body, along with carbonic acid. Metabolic alkalosis and metabolic acidosis may occur due to the deficiency of bicarbonate ions.

Renal, respiratory, and buffer mechanisms maintain the plasma pH at 7.4, carbon dioxide's partial pressure (pCO_2) at 40mm Hg, and the bicarbonate concentration in the plasma around 22-30mmol/liter. The **bicarbonate-carbonic acid system** (the most significant buffer system) operates on a compensatory basis for regulating the acid-base balance.

The main acidic product of metabolism, i.e., the carbonic acid exists in an equilibrium with carbon dioxide and water in body fluids. These in turn are in equilibrium with bicarbonate and hydrogen ions as shown in the following equation:

$$H_2CO_3 \leftrightarrow H_2O + CO_2 \leftrightarrow H^+ + HCO_3^-$$

Functions:

1. Metabolic acidosis (arising from several disorders like diarrhea, diabetic ketoacidosis) and kidney disturbances are treated with sodium bicarbonate due to its alkaline nature.
2. The acid-base balance is maintained by the bicarbonate ion.

4. Sodium: The main extracellular cation is the sodium (Na^+) which is essential for maintaining the osmotic pressure and normal hydration.

Daily diet of a normal human contains more than sufficient amount of sodium which undergoes complete absorption through the intestinal and urinary tract. Kidneys are the vital regulator of sodium concentration in body because excess sodium is excreted by them. The glomerular filtrate reabsorbs 80-85% of sodium which is controlled hormonally; however, this control has not been understood completely.

Daily Requirement: The daily requirement of sodium by an adult is about 2-5gm/day.

Dietary Sources: Sodium can be obtained from foods rich in sodium, like salt, buttermilk, cheese, fish, olives, pulses, etc.

Functions:

1. Osmotic pressure of body fluids is maintained by the sodium ions.
2. Maintaining the cell's osmotic pressure at constant level is the chief function of sodium pump.
3. Acid-base equilibrium is regulated by sodium ions in association with bicarbonate and chloride.
4. Cell's permeability and muscle's irritability are preserved by sodium ions.
5. Glucose absorption by cells for carrying out smooth transportations of nutrients in cell membranes is maintained by sodium ions.
6. Heart's normal functioning is maintained by sodium. It not only maintains the heart contraction of human body, but also the blood pressure levels.

5. Potassium: The major intracellular cation present in the body is potassium (K) whose concentration in intracellular fluid compartment is 23 times higher than that in the extracellular fluid compartment.

Potassium ions along with sodium ions are involved in nerve conduction through **sodium-potassium pump**. There is rapid excretion of excess potassium by the kidney.

Daily Requirement: The daily requirement of potassium by an adult is about 3.5gm/day.

Dietary Sources: Potassium can be obtained from foods rich in potassium, like apricots, bananas, oranges, etc.

Functions:

1. Nerve impulse transmission is regulated by potassium.
2. Many biological activities occurring within the body cells require potassium, **e.g.,** muscle contraction (especially cardiac muscle contractions).
3. Various body fluids' electrolyte composition is maintained by potassium
4. The pH regulation by hydrogen ions exchange is done by potassium ions
5. Treatment and prevention of hypokalemia and/or potassium depletion is done with potassium salts.
6. Restoration in adipose tissue, kidney, Na/K-ATPase, muscle, protein synthesis (on ribosome), erythrocyte (activates pyruvate kinase), and acetylcholine synthesis is done by potassium.
7. Cell's osmotic pressure is also controlled by potassium.

6. Calcium: An important constituent of teeth and bones is calcium (Ca^{2+}) which is involved in muscle functioning and in the blood clotting mechanisms.

Calcium in higher amount is essential in children for growth and development of bones and tissues. Calcium is also stored in bones. In case of intake of calcium deficient diet, the blood calcium level is maintained by bone re-absorption.

Body's 99% calcium content is stored in the bones and the remaining 1% is found in the extracellular fluid compartments. Active transport mechanism helps in the maintenance of this concentration differential.

Total Body Content: 22gm/kg body weight of calcium is present in a human body. **Daily Requirement:** The daily requirement of calcium in an adult human is about 0.8gm/day.

Dietary Sources: Calcium can be obtained from milk, cheese, green vegetables, eggs, and fish.

Functions:

1. Ca^{2+} participates in blood coagulation.
2. Normal cardiac functions are maintained by calcium.
3. Calcium ions play an important role in neuromuscular system and in mechanism of excitation-contraction coupling of the muscles.
4. For the maintenance of mucosal membranes' integrity, individual cell membranes functioning and cell adhesion Ca^{2+} are required.

5. Autonomic nervous system and voluntary systems require calcium ions for their normal functioning.
6. Formation of bones and teeth is carried out by calcium.
7. Formation of solid skeletal material (skulls and bones) in various organisms is done with the help of calcium.
8. Proteins conformation is stabilized with the help of calcium. This role is played by the Ca in DNase, microbial proteinase, and a-amylase.

7. Magnesium: An important intracellular cation is magnesium (Mg^{2+}). Half amount of the body's total magnesium content (around 10-20gm) is combined with phosphorus and calcium in the bone.

Large numbers of enzymes are activated by magnesium, especially carboxylases and kinases. DNA and RNA are also stabilized by magnesium and it is the body's fourth most abundant cation.

Total Body Content: 25gm/kg body weight is the total magnesium content in human body.

Daily Requirement: The daily requirement of magnesium by an adult is about 270-350mg/day.

Dietary Sources: Magnesium can be obtained from foods rich in magnesium, like nuts, un-milled grains, and green vegetables.

Functions:

1. For enzymes that transfer phosphate (PO), magnesium acts as a co-factor.

2. For smooth functioning of neuromuscular system and for protein synthesis, magnesium is used.

3. Teeth and bones essentially constitute magnesium.

4. Glucose metabolism

Q.5. Write a note on Role of Physiological Ions.

Physiological Ions: Body fluids are found in the form of solutions of organic and inorganic solutes. To maintain homeostasis, all the tissues and cells of body continuously try to maintain the concentration of various components.

An ionic balance exists in the solution of each compartment of the body. Therefore, the extracellular fluid (plasma and interstitial fluids) have sodium and chloride ions, whereas, the intracellular fluid has magnesium, phosphate (as phosphate esters, HPO_4^{2-} and $H_2PO_4^{2-}$) and potassium ions.

Following are the **major physiological ions**:

1. Chloride,
2. Phosphate,
3. Bicarbonate,
4. Sodium,
5. Potassium,
6. Calcium, and
7. Magnesium

Role of Physiological Ions: Role of physiological ions in body are as follows:

1. These ions participate in nerve conduction (sodium and potassium are involved in nerve conduction) and muscle contraction.

   Example: Calcium is involved in muscle contraction.

2. Various enzymes and coenzymes are activated by reacting with physiological ions.

   Example: kinase enzyme is activated by combining to magnesium.

3. Physiological ions are major part of electrolyte replacement therapy.

4. Dialysis fluid is prepared by combining various physiological ions indifferent concentrations.

5. Physiological ions (e.g., carbonates, bicarbonates, etc.) are directly involved in regulation of acid and bases.

Q.6. Discuss Electrolytes Used in Replacement Therapy with example.

Electrolytes Replacement Therapy: To maintain the homeostasis, concentration of electrolytes in the body fluids should also be constant. However, the electrolyte balance in the body is disturbed in cases when an individual remains ill for a long duration or undergoes surgery or remains under prolonged unfavorable conditions. Electrolyte imbalances due to such reasons are corrected or maintained by the replacement therapy in which electrolytes are administered externally.

Basic objective of replacement therapy is to restore and maintain the composition and volume of body fluid. Decrease in volume of body fluids may be a life-threatening condition, as it causes impairment in circulation. As a result, a decrease in blood volume and fall in cardiac output is observed due to which the microcirculation integrity gets adversely affected.

The various mechanisms of the body under normal physiological conditions maintain the electrolyte balance, and thus, there is no need of replacement therapy in a healthy person. However, there may be severe water and electrolytes loss in conditions like prolonged fever, vomiting, trauma, etc.

There are usually **three types of solutions** used in the replacement therapy:

1. Sodium potassium replacement,
2. Parenteral magnesium administration, and
3. Calcium replacement.

1. Sodium and Potassium Replacement: Sodium (Na) is a chief electrolyte and forms a part of many replenishment products. Sodium replenishment is based on electrolyte replenishment as it contains unique combination of ingredients that could restore the loss of sodium ion during an exercise process. To achieve this goal, it is necessary o activate the transport systems by proper addition of alanine and zinc. This results in the complete and rapid replenishment of an electrolyte as compared to the traditional salt.

In our body, potassium is the **major intracellular cation**. It also helps to regulate muscular contraction as well as neuromuscular excitability.

For therapeutic purposes, potassium salts act as an essential component, but when used improperly it may be toxic. Kidneys play a vital role in absorption and secretion of potassium ion. However, aldosterone helps to enhance the reabsorption of sodium as well as the secretion of potassium by kidneys. For these purposes' kidney absorbs potassium of body tissues, mainly from tissues of the liver and muscles.

Excess depletion of potassium involves increased excretion of it by kidney and GIT. The main **causes of renal excretion of potassium** are

- ➤ Diuretic therapy
- ➤ Large doses of anionic drugs, and
- ➤ Renal disorders

Examples of potassium and sodium replenisher are:

1. Sodium chloride (NaCl),
2. Potassium chloride (KCl),
3. Compound sodium chloride solution (lactated Ringer's solution).
4. Oral rehydration solution (ORS), etc.

Sodium Chloride (NaCl): Sodium chloride (mol. wt. 58.44) contains not more than 99.5% of NaCl; none other constituents are added in it.

Naturally, it is present in sea water, lakes (Sambhar in India, Lake Elton in Russia), in salt wells, and deposits of nock salt (in Punjab, Pakistan).

Method of Preparation:

Commercially, sodium chloride is prepared from shallow pans of seawater by the process of evaporation. It contains several impurities such as sodium carbonate, sodium sulphate, magnesium chloride, magnesium sulphate, and calcium chloride. For removal of impurities, firstly, the common salt is to be dissolved in the cemented tanks, and then some lime and alum are added as a result, the suspended impurities start settling down and then the clear solutions are poured into iron pans. Solution is concentrated and crystals of sodium chloride are separated after they settle down. Finally, the saturated solution is pumped out and converted into salt by the process of evaporation.

Assay:

Around 0.1gm of sample is dissolved in 50ml of water. Thereafter, 1ml of 0.1N $AgNO_3$ 3ml HNO_3, 5ml nitro-benzene, and 2ml of ferric ammonium sulphate are added in 50ml of water. The resultant solution is titrated with0.1N ammonium thiocyanate until it changes to reddish yellow in color.

1ml of 0.1N $AgNO_3$ ≡ 0.005844gm NaCl

Physical Properties:

1. Appearance: Colorless or white crystalline solid
2. Crystal Structure: Cubic
3. Odor: Odorless
4. Specific Gravity: 2.16
5. pH: 6.7-7.3 (aqueous solution)
6. Melting Point: 801°C
7. Boiling Point: 1413°C
8. Stability: Stable under ordinary conditions of use and storage
9. Solubility: Freely soluble in water; slightly more soluble in boiling water, soluble in glycerin; slightly soluble in alcohol.

Chemical Properties:

1. It gives a curd-like white precipitate by reacting with silver nitrate solution.

$$NaCl + AgNO_3 \rightarrow AgCl \downarrow + NaNO_3$$

2. It oxidizes to give chlorine when heated with concentrated sulphuric acid and magnesium dioxide.

$$2NaCl + MnO_2 + 2H_2SO_4 \rightarrow MnSO_4 + Na_2SO_4 + 2H_2O + Cl_2 \uparrow$$

3. It produces hydrochloric acid by reacting with sulphuric acid.

$$2NaCl + H_2SO_4 \rightarrow 2HCl + Na_2SO_4$$

Medicinal Uses:

1. It is used in the treatment of dehydration, sodium depletion, volume depletion which may result due to:

    (I) Excessive diuresis,

(II) Gastroenteritis, and

(III) Salt restriction.

2. A 0.9% of sodium chloride salt solution is used:

   (I) As eye-drops (as an irritating agent),

   (II) As nasal drop (to relieve nasal congestion), and

   (III) As a mouthwash (to remove debris, for throat infection).

3. It is also added in dermatological preparations as a hydrating agent.

4. It is also used in the preparation of some formulations.

2. Parenteral Magnesium Administration: Magnesium is the fourth most abundant cation in the human body after sodium, potassium, and calcium. It is the second most common cation in intracellular fluid.

The normal human body contains 21-28gm of magnesium, approximately 53% in bones, 27% in muscles, 19% in non- muscular soft tissues, and only 1% in extracellular fluid. Normal serum magnesium concentrations range from 1.6-2.6mg/dL.

Magnesium is one of the chief constituents of many biochemical compounds. It participates in many metabolic processes and can be involved in many **functions** such as:

1. Production of energy

2. Storage

3. Utilization of ATP, and

4. Some enzymatic reactions involved in protein synthesis

Some other **essential uses of magnesium** are:

1. Neuromuscular transmission
2. Cardiac excitability
3. Cardiovascular tone, and
4. Control of neuronal activity

Concentration of magnesium is mainly controlled by kidney; in case of deficiency of magnesium, kidneys conserve the remaining magnesium. In case of higher concentration of magnesium, it can be easily expelled through urine.

The most common magnesium replenishers are:

1. Magnesium chloride,
2. Magnesium sulphate, etc.

3. Calcium Replacement: Calcium is a metal with stable cation and it is relatively reactive in nature. However, with soluble carbonates, oxalates, sulphates, borates, citrates, phosphates, and tartrates, calcium in soluble form undergoes metathesis (exchange of cations and anions) and yields calcium compounds of insoluble matter. Pharmaceutical incompatibilities are generated due to such reactions.

Calcium along with magnesium constitutes 98% mass of teeth and bones. Many physiological processes use calcium as a vital part. Representation of some therapeutic categories is done with the help of official calcium compounds. These include calcium replenishers and the antacids.

In order to carry the therapeutically active anions, calcium is mostly the choice in the form of cations, calcium cyclobarbital and calcium amino salicylate.

Examples of calcium replenishers:

1. Calcium gluconate,
2. Calcium chloride,
3. Calcium lactate,
4. Calcium levulinate, etc.

Calcium gluconate: Calcium gluconate (mol. wt. 430.38) is the calcium salt of gluconic acid containing 9% of calcium ions (Ca^{2+}). Calcium gluconate has many applications, but most commonly it is used in hypocalcaemia as a calcium replenisher.

Methods of Preparation:

Gluconic acid solution is heated with calcium carbonate (slight excess). The resultant mixture is filtered and the filtrate is crystallized to obtain calcium gluconate crystals.

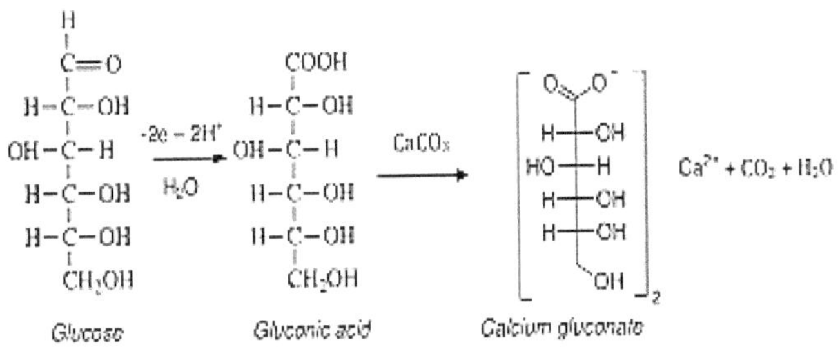

Glucose   Gluconic acid   Calcium gluconate

Assay: The complexometric titration method is used in the assay of calcium gluconate and other calcium salts. A stable complex is formed by calcium ions with EDTA disodium salt.

This sample is treated with hydrochloric acid and its pH is maintained (around 10) by adding a buffer solution of strong ammonia and ammonium chloride. The resultant solution is titrated against standard disodium edetate solution and mordant black II mixture is used as an indicator.

$$Ca^{++} + Na_2H_2V \rightarrow Na_2CaV + 2H^+$$
$$C_{12}H_{22}O_{14}H_2O \equiv Na_2H_2V \equiv Ca^{++}$$
$$= 1000ml\ 1M\ Na_2H_2V$$

1000ml of 1M Monosodium edetate $\equiv$ **44.8gm of** $CaC_{12}H_{22}O_{14}.H_2O$
Each ml of 0.50M Monosodium edetate $\equiv$ **0.2242gm of** $CaC_{12}H_{22}O_{14}H_2O$

Procedure:

1. 0.8gm of calcium gluconate is weighed.
2. This calcium gluconate is dissolved in 150ml of water containing previously added 5ml of dilute hydrochloric acid.
3. About 15ml of a buffer of strong ammonia and ammonium chloride is then added.
4. The resultant solution is later titrated with 0.05M disodium edetate using 40mg of mordant black II as an indicator, until the solution turns deep blue in colour.

   In order to make the end point sharp, 5ml of 0.05M magnesium sulphate solution is generally added before the titration.

Physical Properties:

1. Appearance: White crystalline powder.
2. Odour: Odorless.
3. Taste: Tasteless.
4. Stability: Stable in air and does not lose its water on drying without undergoing decomposition.
5. Solubility: Soluble in water (1gm in 30ml); insoluble in alcohol.
6. pH: Its solutions are neutral to litmus paper.

Chemical Properties:

1. It shows incompatibility with Oxidising agents. It undergoes precipitation with borate, oxalate, etc.
2. It undergoes decomposition with dilute mineral acids.

Medicinal Uses:

1. It can be administered orally as it is less irritating than calcium chloride.
2. It is a source of Ca^{2+} that is readily available. Severe **hypocalcemia tetany** can be treated by giving this salt intravenously.
3. It is either applied topically as a gel or injected as a solution for treating the burns caused by hydrofluoric acid.

Q.7. Give the preparation, Properties, Assay and uses of Sodium Chloride and Calcium Gluconate.

SODIUM CHLORIDE (NaCl): Sodium chloride (mol. wt. 58.44) contains not more than 99.5% of NaCl; none other constituents are added in it. Naturally, it is present in sea water, lakes (Sambhar in India, Lake Elton in Russia), in salt wells, and deposits of nock salt (in Punjab, Pakistan).

Method of Preparation:

Commercially, sodium chloride is prepared from shallow pans of seawater by the process of evaporation. It contains several impurities such as sodium carbonate, sodium sulphate, magnesium chloride, magnesium sulphate, and calcium chloride. For removal of impurities, firstly, the common salt is to be dissolved in the cemented tanks, and then some lime and alum are added as a result, the suspended impurities start settling down and then the clear solutions are poured into iron pans. Solution is concentrated and crystals of sodium chloride are separated after they settle down. Finally, the saturated solution is pumped out and converted into salt by the process of evaporation.

Assay: Around 0.1gm of sample is dissolved in 50ml of water. Thereafter, 1ml of 0.1N $AgNO_3$ 3ml HNO_3, 5ml nitro-benzene, and 2ml of ferric ammonium sulphate are added in 50ml of water. The resultant solution is titrated with0.1N ammonium thiocyanate until it changes to reddish yellow in color.

1ml of 0.1N $AgNO_3$ ≡ 0.005844gm NaCl

Physical Properties:

1. Appearance: Colorless or white crystalline solid

2. Crystal Structure: Cubic

3. Odor: Odorless

4. Specific Gravity: 2.16

5. pH: 6.7-7.3 (aqueous solution)

6. Melting Point: 801°C

7. Boiling Point: 1413°C

8. Stability: Stable under ordinary conditions of use and storage

9. Solubility: Freely soluble in water; slightly more soluble in boiling water, soluble in glycerin; slightly soluble in alcohol.

Chemical Properties:

1. It gives a curd-like white precipitate by reacting with silver nitrate solution.

$$NaCl + AgNO_3 \rightarrow AgCl \downarrow + NaNO3$$

2. It oxidizes to give chlorine when heated with concentrated sulphuric acid and magnesium dioxide.

$$2NaCl + MnO_2 + 2H_2SO_4 \rightarrow MnSO_4 + Na_2SO_4 + 2H_2O + Cl_2 \uparrow$$

3. It produces hydrochloric acid by reacting with sulphuric acid.

$$2NaCl + H_2SO_4 \rightarrow 2HCl + Na_2SO_4$$

Medicinal Uses:

1. It is used in the treatment of dehydration, sodium depletion, volume depletion which may result due to:

   (I)   Excessive diuresis,

(II)   Gastroenteritis, and

(III)   Salt restriction.

2. A 0.9% of sodium chloride salt solution is used:

(I)   As eye-drops (as an irritating agent),

(II)   As nasal drop (to relieve nasal congestion), and

(III)   As a mouthwash (to remove debris, for throat infection).

3. It is also added in dermatological preparations as a hydrating agent.

4. It is also used in the preparation of some formulations.

CALCIUM GLUCONATE: Calcium gluconate (mol. wt. 430.38) is the calcium salt of gluconic acid containing 9% of calcium ions (Ca^{2+}). Calcium gluconate has many applications, but most commonly it is used in hypocalcaemia as a calcium replenisher.

Glucose   Gluconic acid   Calcium gluconate

Methods of Preparation: Gluconic acid solution is heated with calcium carbonate (slight excess). The resultant mixture is filtered and the filtrate is crystallized to obtain calcium gluconate crystals.

Assay: The complexometric titration method is used in the assay of calcium gluconate and other calcium salts. A stable complex is formed by calcium ions with EDTA disodium salt.

This sample is treated with hydrochloric acid and its pH is maintained (around 10) by adding a buffer solution of strong ammonia and ammonium chloride. The resultant solution is titrated against standard disodium edetate solution and mordant black II mixture is used as an indicator.

$$Ca^{++} + Na_2H_2V \rightarrow Na_2CaV + 2H^+$$
$$C_{12}H_{22}O_{14}H_2O \equiv Na_2H_2V \equiv Ca^{++}$$
$$= 1000ml\ 1M\ Na_2H_2V$$

1000ml of 1M Monosodium edetate $\equiv$ 44.8gm of $CaC_{12}H_{22}O_{14}.H_2O$
Each ml of 0.50M Monosodium edetate $\equiv$ 0.2242gm of $CaC_{12}H_{22}O_{14}H_2O$

Procedure:

1. 0.8gm of calcium gluconate is weighed.

2. This calcium gluconate is dissolved in 150ml of water containing previously added 5ml of dilute hydrochloric acid.

3. About 15ml of a buffer of strong ammonia and ammonium chloride is then added.

4. The resultant solution is later titrated with 0.05M disodium edetate using 40mg of mordant black II as an indicator, until the solution turns deep blue in colour.

   In order to make the end point sharp, 5ml of 0.05M magnesium sulphate solution is generally added before the titration.

Physical Properties:

1. Appearance: White crystalline powder.
2. Odour: Odourless.

3. Taste: Tasteless.

4. Stability: Stable in air and does not lose its water on drying without undergoing decomposition.

5. Solubility: Soluble in water (1gm in 30ml); insoluble in alcohol.

6. pH: Its solutions are neutral to litmus paper.

Chemical Properties:

1. It shows incompatibility with oxidising agents. It undergoes precipitation with borate, oxalate, etc.

2. It undergoes decomposition with dilute mineral acids.

Medicinal Uses:

1. It can be administered orally as it is less irritating than calcium chloride.

2. It is a source of Ca^{2+} that is readily available. Severe **hypocalcemia tetany** can be treated by giving this salt intravenously.

3. It is either applied topically as a gel or injected as a solution for treating the burns caused by hydrofluoric acid.

Q.8. Give the Preparation, Properties and Uses of Potassium Chloride.

Potassium Chloride (KCl): Potassium chloride (molecular weight 74.56) contains not more than 99.5% of KCl, calculated with reference to the substance dried at constant temperature of 105°C for 2 hours.

Methods of Preparation:

1. The salt is mainly obtained from cornallite (KEL.MgCl2.6H_2O) and is usually found as sylvine. The crushed cornallite is warmed at suitable temperature with liquor having magnesium chloride. Then the magnesium chloride and potassium chloride are dissolved in cornallite. After an hour, undissolved material starts settling down, and the hot liquid is decanted to cool. Crude potassium chloride starts depositing and recrystallizing.

2. In laboratory, it can be prepared by treating HCl with bicarbonates or potassium carbonate.

$$K_2CO_3 + 2HCl \rightarrow 2KCl + H_2O + CO_2 \uparrow$$
$$KHCO_3 + HCl \rightarrow KCl + H_2O + CO_2 \uparrow$$

Physical Properties:

1. Appearance: Crystalline white solid.
2. Crystal Structure: Cubic.
3. Solubility: Less soluble in water than sodium chloride; soluble in glycerin and ether.
4. Odour: Odourless.
5. Taste: Saline.
6. Melting Point: 772°C.
7. pH: Its 10% aqueous solution is neutral to litmus paper.

Chemical Properties: Chemically, chloride can be precipitated by some ions (such as Ag^+, Hg^{2+} and Pb^2) in the qualitative analysis.

Medicinal Uses:

1. The salt is employed for the **oral replacement of potassium** in the form of solution. Sometimes, this aqueous solution can also create irritation in the gastrointestinal tract. It can be administered intravenously, if not given orally or in the condition of hypokalaemia.

2. It is given in treatment of cardiac arrhythmia, especially when myocardium cells are depleted of potassium ions.

3. It is also used in the treatment of periodic paralysis and Meniere's **syndrome** (disease of inner ear).

4. It is also used to cure mental disorder, and **myasthenia gravis** (severe muscular weakness).

Q.9. Discuss Renal Replacement Therapy (Dialysis Fluid).

Dialysis Fluids: Dialysis is a **renal replacement therapy**, useful when kidneys stop functioning due to damage or failure. In dialysis, functions performed by the kidneys are replaced artificially. Very sick patients who are suffering from acute renal failure or have suddenly lost their kidney function temporarily may undergo dialysis. It may also be used for patients who are stable but their kidney function is lost permanently.

Electrolyte solutions which are circulated across permeable membranes to carry out the exchange of electrolytes, fluids and other chemicals from and to the body fluids are termed as dialysis fluids.

The dialysis fluids are not meant for internal administration; therefore, their concentration is similar to that of extracellular fluids.

Types of Dialysis fluids:

1. Haemodialysis fluids
2. Peritoneal dialysis fluids

1. Haemodialysis Fluids: Large quantities of these fluids are used along with the artificial kidney machine.

A tank is used to keep the haemodialysis fluid from which it is agitated constantly and is circulated to the patient's blood across a synthetic semi-permeable membrane using a bypass system.

Exchange of ions and glucose takes place across the semi-permeable membrane, thus, achieving a state of equilibrium.

The waste products (urea) and other chemicals to be excreted also passes into the dialysis fluid at the same time.

Final Diluted Haemodialysis Solution

Sodium	130-140mmol/L
Potassium	0-3mmol/L
Calcium	1-2mmol/L
Magnesium	0.25-1.0mmol/L
Acetate or lactate (expressed as bicarbonate)	32-40mmol/L
Chloride	95-110mmol/L

Peritoneal dialysis fluids:

Sodium Chloride	5.56gm
Magnesium Chloride	0.152gm
Sodium Acetate	4.76gm
Calcium Chloride	0.22gm
Sodium Metabisulphate	0.15gm
Dextrose (anhydrous)	17.0gm
Purified water	q.s.

Q.10. What is Physiological Acid-Base Balance? Give brief Mechanism involved in Acid-Base Balance.

Physiological Acid-Base Balance: A human body has mainly **three main control systems** that are used for the following purposes:

1. To maintain acid-base balance in alkalosis or acidosis condition,
2. In the buffer systems,
3. Respirations, and
4. Renal control of H' ion.

Acidity of a solution indicates the presence of a acidity total H^+ ion found in a of solution. Hence, the pH can be defined as the total measurement in the solution or the negative logarithm of H^+ ion.

In body fluids, acids and bases are found in an appropriate amount. The concentration of acids and bases should be maintained because the biochemical reactions occur in body are very sensitive even to a change in the alkalinity or acidity.

The pH of blood in normal healthy person is approximately 7.35. Low pH of blood indicates high hydrogen ion concentration leading to acidosis. At high pH, this shows the presence of less hydrogen ions resulting in slight alkalosis. The normal pH of human beings ranges from 7.0-7.8.

Mechanism of Acid-Base Balance: Several mechanisms that help to maintain the acid-base balance of the bodyare as follows:

1. **Buffer System:** A weak acid and its salt (that functions like a weak base) can together act as a buffer system. Body's buffer system resist pH to change rapidly as it converts the strong bases and acids into weak bases and acids. Therefore, removing the excess hydrogen ions not from the body but only from the body fluids.

   In the body fluids, the following major buffer systems exist:

   i. Carbonic Acid-Bicarbonate Buffer System: This buffer system, existing in kidneys and plasma is an essential blood pH regulator. Bicarbonate (HCO_3^-) ion forms carbonic acid by acting as a weak base and accepting H ions that are present in in the body fluids. The carbonic acid further undergoes dissociation to produce water, along with carbon dioxide.

   $$H^+ + HCO_3^- \rightarrow H_2CO_3 \rightarrow H_2O + CO_2$$

Strong acid	**weak base**	**Carbonic acid**
(weak acid)		

However, carbonic acid (another component of the buffer system) maintains the pH by undergoing ionization and producing more hydrogen ions when present in low concentration.

$$H_2CO_3 \rightarrow H^+ + HCO_3^-$$

For example, oxygen in lungs releases protons by reacting with the protonated deoxy haemoglobin. These released protons form carbonic acid on combining with the bicarbonate ion. The carbonic acid formed further undergoes dissociation to yield water, along with carbon dioxide which will be exhaled.

ii. **Phosphate Buffer System:** This buffer system also maintains the blood pH at 7.4. It acts as a cytosol pH regulator because the concentration of phosphate is highest in the intracellular fluid. The HPO_4^{2-} /$H_2PO_4^-$ (mono hydrogen phosphate/dihydrogen phosphate) anions are present in this system. In cells and kidneys, these act the carbonic acid-bicarbonate buffer system.

Monohydrogen phosphate ion acts as a weak base and accepts proton when excess of H^+ ions are present in the body fluids.

$$HCl + Na_2HPO_4 \rightarrow NaCl + NaH_2PO_4$$

On the other hand, dihydrogen phosphate ion acts as a weak acid and causes neutralization of alkaline condition.

$$NaOH + NaH_2PO_4 \rightarrow H_2O + Na_2HPO_4$$

For example, if excess of hydrogen ion (present in the kidney tubules) combines with Na_2HPO_4, formation of NaH_2PO_4 in kidneys occur. This reaction results in the production of Na^+ ions which combine with bicarbonate ion to form sodium bicarbonate which enters the blood.

iii. **Protein (Haemoglobin) Buffer System:** This buffer system is abundantly found in body plasma and cells. Amino acids possessing at least one amino group (NH_2) and one carboxyl group (COOH) combine to form proteins. The amino group in the presence of excess hydrogen ions accepts protons by acting as a base.

$$HOOC{-}RCH{-}NH_2 + H^+ \rightarrow HOOC{-}RCH{-}NH_3$$

The alkaline conditions are neutralized by the protons released by the free carboxyl group. Thus, proteins being amphoteric act as both the acidic and basic components of a buffer system. Cysteines and histidine's are the most vital amino acid buffers at physiological pH. Haemoglobin, effectively acts as a physiological buffer as it is a protein, structurally made up of 37 histidine's.

The pH of the body fluids is also maintained by **breathing**.

$$CO_2 + H_2O \leftrightarrow H_2CO_3 \leftrightarrow H^+HCO_3$$

Pharmaceutical Inorganic Chemistry More carbon dioxide will be exhaled when breathing depth and rate increases, thus, decreasing H_2CO_3 formation rate which ultimately decreases the hydrogen ion concentration. As a result, body fluid's pH is also increased. On the other hand, less carbon dioxide is exhaled when the respiration rate slows down, thus, decreasing the pH of blood.

2. **Elimination of Some Ions through Urine by Kidney:** Certain ions are absorbed and other are eliminated through body fluids, thus, maintaining the acid-base balance of blood, as well as the body fluids.

3. **Through Respiratory Centre:** Control of respiratory center helps in controlling the pH. Breathing rate is altered as a result of the stimulation of respiratory center. This change occurring in the breathing rate controls the carbon dioxide removal from body fluids, thus, changing the pH of carbonic acid in blood.

Q.11. Write an exhaustive note on Electrolyte Combination Therapy.

Electrolyte Combination Therapy: After surgery the patient is kept under some short-term therapies to fulfil the essential body requirements as he/she is not able to intake normal or balanced diet. Such short-term therapy includes infusions comprising of saline and glucose. While, a complete **electrolyte combination therapy** is used for the treatment of patients suffering from chronic illness or severe loss of fluid. For this purpose, combination of electrolytes is given to patient for the maintenance of body fluids.

Electrolyte combination products are divided into two basic categories:

1. Fluid maintenance, and
2. Electrolyte replacement.

A number of electrolyte combinations (of varying compositions) available in the market either in the form of **dry powders** which can be dissolved in water (specified quantity), or as prepared solutions, known as **oral electrolyte solutions**.

Both sucrose and starch exert glucose-like effect in the intestine. Under **Oral Rehydration Therapy (ORT)** a fluid containing a suitable combination of carbohydrates and electrolytes is given through oral route.

The composition of carbohydrate-electrolyte mixtures of ORT vary significantly in sodium content. This therapy is beneficial for controlling the possibilities of death due to diarrhoea. The easiest way, of preparing ORT solution is to prepare a solution of sugar and salt.

Oral Rehydration Solution (ORS): Oral rehydration solutions are given to the patients to prevent or treat mild to moderate fluid loss (5-10% dehydration) resulted due to diarrhoea or postoperative conditions or when food and liquid intake have been stopped momentarily. ORS provides sodium, chloride, potassium, water and other basic nutrients. Sodium transport and water absorption are carried out by a carbohydrate (2-2.5% glucose) present in it.

ORS Composition: The standard (310mOsm/L) ORS formula has been replaced by the new (245mOsm/L) formula of ORS as per the recommendations of WHO and UNICEF.

New Formula WHO-ORS

Composition	Amount	Ions	Concentration
NaCl	2.6g	Na^+	75mM
KCl	1.5gm	K^+	20mM
Trisodium citrate	2.9gm	Cl^-	65mM
Glucose	13.5gm	Citrate	10mM
Water	1L	Glucose	75mM
Total osmolarity 245mOsm/L			

In most of the cases of acute diarrhoea, it has been seen that large amounts of K^+ are lost; therefore, potassium is the chief constituent of ORS. Bases, **e.g.,** bicarbonate, citrate, etc. are added in ORS to correct the conditions of acidosis (condition in which excessive loss of alkali occurs in stools). It can also promote sodium and water absorption.

Administration: Patients are suggested to drink ORS at regular intervals of 1/2-1hour. In the beginning. 5-7.5% volume is given in every 2-4 hours. Feeling of thirst arises due to volume depletion, thus, it can be effective to control the loss in stools. If a physically weak child refuses to drink ORS, it can be given through intragastric drip, with an aim to restore the hydration within 6 hours.

Adverse Effects:

1. Hypernatremia (condition in which the sodium level in blood is elevated),
2. Hyperkalaemia (condition in which the concentration of electrolyte potassium is elevated), and

3. Acid-base disturbances occurring occasionally.

All these conditions are seen in case of renal failure or if errors occur reforming the bulk powders.

Contraindications:

1. Repeated vomiting,
2. Dynamic ileus (condition caused by inhibition of bowel motility),
3. Perforated bowel,
4. Shock,
5. Renal dysfunction, and
6. Monosaccharide malabsorption.

Precautions:

1. Parenteral replacement therapy is used to maintain electrolyte imbalances that has occurred due to fluid loss (10-15% of the body weight), inability to take fluids, severe gastric distension, or severe vomiting.
2. Errors in rebuilding or diluting the viable powders.

Uses: ORS is preferred to maintain the level of electrolytes in case of severe fluid loss, and severe gastric swelling. In case of inability to take fluids in food, and severe vomiting, parenteral replacement therapy is used.

Oral Rehydration Therapy (ORT): ORT a simple, cheap and effective therapy used for treating dehydration caused by diarrhoea or gastroenteritis (caused by cholera or rotavirus).

ORT comprises of a solution of salt and sugars taken orally. It is being used all over the world, but mainly in developing countries, where it has saved millions of children's life suffering from diarrhoea.

Uses:

1. Infectious diarrhoeas,
2. Short bowel syndrome,
3. Diarrhoeal illness in nursing home residents,
4. Paediatric viral illnesses,
5. AIDS, and
6. Salt wasting nephropathies.

Disadvantages:

1. The volume, frequency, or duration of diarrhoea are not affected by them,
2. Expensive,
3. Less nutritional value, and
4. Unpleasant taste.

Q.12. What is ORS? Give their formula.

Oral Rehydration Solution (ORS): Oral rehydration solutions are given to the patients to prevent or treat mild to moderate fluid loss (5-10% dehydration) resulted due to diarrhoea or postoperative conditions or when food and liquid intake have been stopped momentarily. ORS provides sodium, chloride, potassium, water and other basic nutrients. Sodium transport and water absorption are carried out by a carbohydrate (2-2.5% glucose) present in it.

New Formula WHO-ORS

Composition	Amount	Ions	Concentration
NaCl	2.6g	Na^+	75mM
KCl	1.5gm	K^+	20mM
Trisodium citrate	2.9gm	Cl^-	65mM
Glucose	13.5gm	Citrate	10mM
Water	1L	Glucose	75mM
Total osmolarity 245mOsm/L			

ORS Composition: The standard (310mOsm/L) ORS formula has been replaced by the new (245mOsm/L) formula of ORS as per the recommendations of WHO and UNICEF.

Administration: Patients are suggested to drink ORS at regular intervals of 1/2-1hour. In the beginning. 5-7.5% volume is given in every 2-4 hours. Feeling of thirst arises due to volume depletion, thus, it can be effective to control the loss in stools. If a physically weak child refuses to drink ORS, it can be given through intragastric drip, with an aim to restore the hydration within 6 hours.

Adverse Effects:

1. Hypernatremia (condition in which the sodium level in blood is elevated),

2. Hyperkalaemia (condition in which the concentration of electrolyte potassium is elevated), and

3. Acid-base disturbances occurring occasionally.

All these conditions are seen in case of renal failure or if errors occur reforming the bulk powders.

Contraindications:

1. Repeated vomiting, Shock,

2. Dynamic ileus (condition caused by inhibition of bowel motility),

3. Perforated bowel,

4. Renal dysfunction, and

5. Monosaccharide malabsorption.

Precautions:

1. Parenteral replacement therapy is used to maintain electrolyte imbalances that has occurred due to fluid loss (10-15% of the body weight), inability to take fluids, severe gastric distension, or severe vomiting.

2. Errors in rebuilding or diluting the viable powders.

Uses: ORS is preferred to maintain the level of electrolytes in case of severe fluid loss, and severe gastric swelling. In case of inability to take fluids in food, and severe vomiting, parenteral replacement therapy is used.

UNIT – 2
2.3. <u>DENTAL PRODUCTS</u>

Q.1. Write a note on Dental Products with Cleaning agents.

Dental Products: Today numerous dental products are available in the market that helps to maintain dental health and hygiene. Various factors have been responsible for dental decay and other dental problems.

In dental decay, various factors have been used due to which oral hygienic problems arise. Numerous inorganic compounds are used in dental products and in dentistry.

These include mainly:

1. Cleaning agents,
2. Dentifrices,
3. Anticaries agents/fluorides,
4. Desensitizing agent,
5. Cements and fillers,
6. Oral antiseptics and astringents, and
7. Polishing/abrasive agents.

Cleaning Agents: An efficient cleaning agent must comprise of fine particles having suitable property. It must provide suitable abrasiveness in order to remove stains from teeth. However, the evaluation of abrasiveness is very difficult. Few tests are proposed to evaluate these cleaning agents but these are not applicable for in vivo studies.

The phosphates are generally used as anticaries and cleaning agents. Few popular cleaning agents used in the preparation of toothpaste and toothpowders are dibasic and tribasic calcium phosphate and sodium meta- phosphate. Other less common cleansing agents are calcium carbonate, pumice powders, etc.

Q.2. Write a note on Dental Products and Describe the role of fluoride as anti-caries agents.

Dental Products: Today numerous dental products are available in the market that helps to maintain dental health and hygiene. Various factors have been responsible for dental decay and other dental problems.

In dental decay, various factors have been used due to which oral hygienic problems arise. Numerous inorganic compounds are used in dental products and in dentistry.

These include mainly:

8. Cleaning agents,
9. Dentifrices,
10. Anticaries agents/fluorides,
11. Desensitizing agent,
12. Cements and fillers,
13. Oral antiseptics and astringents, and
14. Polishing/abrasive agents.

Anticaries Agents/Fluorides: When act on carbohydrates, acids are produced which causes dental caries or tooth decay, i.e., decalcification of tooth, along with foul mouth odour.

Role of Fluoride in the Treatment of Dental Caries: Fluoride is generally added in dentifrices to prevent dental caries. Outstanding results are obtained when trace amount of fluoride salts is applied topically to the teeth.

In human body, fluoride ion is present in trace amount and sufficient quantity is usually obtained from food and water. But places where ground water is lacking in fluoride element, dental problems (like dental caries) are more common and prevalent.

The process of adding fluoride to the municipal water supply is termed as **fluoridation**. This is generally performed to reduce and prevent dental caries. However, slow continued ingestion of fluoride may result in teeth mottling, increased bone density, gastric disturbances, muscular weakness, convulsions, and even heart failure. But, due to its effectiveness in treating dental caries and other types of osteoporosis, fluorides are frequently used in dental practice.

The fluorides can be administered either through oral or topical route. After the internal administration of fluoride salt or solution, it is rapidly absorbed, transported and deposited in the bone or developing teeth. The remaining concentration of fluorides is excreted through kidneys.

The fluoride deposited on the surface of teeth is required to prevent dental carries and is also required to avoid the occurrence of lesions on the teeth surfaces due to action of acids or enzymes. A small quantity of fluoride (1ppm) is usually added in the preparation, whereas more quantity of fluoride (more than 2-3ppm) may cause mottling of teeth enamel and is usually known as **dental fluorosis**.

The fluoridation of public water supply is the most common and efficient means of oral administration. Usually 0.5-1ppm of fluoride salts are added in the water supply. It should be added to drinking water or fruit juice in concentration not more than 1ppm per day.

About 2.2mg of sodium fluoride tablets or solution are used per day. Approximately 2% solution of fluoride is applied topically over teeth.

Fluorides either work by **reducing the ability of bacteria to make acids** or by **re-mineralizing the areas of the tooth** that have been attacked by acids from bacteria.

Mechanism of Action: The fluoride ion (F^-) is known to **replace the hydroxyl ion (OH^-) in hydroxyl apatite**, which is the main crystalline structure of enamel. The replaced crystal is known as **fluorapatite** which is more resistant to acids produced by plaque bacteria than the hydroxyl apatite. The absorption of fluoride into enamel can be illustrated through the following chemical reaction:

$$Ca_{10}(PO_4)_6(OH)_2 + 2F^- \rightarrow Ca_{10}(PO_4)_6F_2 + 2(OH)^-$$

Fluoride is an anti-enzyme and generally inhibits the activity of enzymatic acid produced by plaque bacteria. However, the tooth develops and enamel is formed, ingested fluoride gets incorporated into the enamel. In comparison to inner layers, more fluoride is required to develop the outer layer of enamel. The fluoride deposited on the surface enamel layer provides protection against caries.

Examples:

1. Sodium fluoride,
2. Sodium metaphosphate,
3. Stannous fluoride, and
4. Zinc chloride.

Q.3. What are dentifrices? Give characteristics, types and example.

Dentifrices: A dentifrice is a substance used for cleaning the reachable surfaces of the teeth with a toothbrush. The main objective of a dentifrice is to help the toothbrush clean the teeth. Brushing of teeth with or without a dentifrice is beneficial to dental health. A dentifrice is used to maintain good oral hygiene.

Toothpaste is the most common dentifrice that dentists recommend to use with a toothbrush for removing dental plaque and food debris.

Characteristics: Dentifrices possess the following characteristics:

1. Flavors and soaps or synthetic detergents, abrasives and antibacterial agents are present in many dentifrices.
2. Fluorides (especially stannous) which are topically effective may also be present in dentifrices. But they are compounded by a different method with polishing agents and surfactants.
3. CaCO3 as a polishing agent is also used in dentifrices.
4. Dentifrices are unable to clean the surfaces within the cavities and crevices between teeth.
5. Abrasive property and the force applied for rubbing influences the cleaning action of dentifrices.
6. **Medicated dentifrices** are also available which contain substances for better oral hygiene and supplying trace materials (e.g., fluoride, antiseptics, deodorants, etc.).

7. **Flavors** and **colors** are added to dentifrices for promoting their acceptance.

8. Dentifrices should be sufficiently abrasive so that they can remove stains from teeth.

9. Phosphate plays a major role as anticaries and dentifrice. Dibasic and tribasic calcium phosphate and sodium metaphosphate are commonly used dentifrices in toothpaste and tooth powders. Similarly, calcium carbonate and pumice powder can also be used as dentifrice agents.

Types: Dentifrices are of three types depending on whether they are solid, semi-solid or liquid:

1. **Toothpaste:** It is used with a toothbrush for maintaining oral hygiene. Toothpaste is mainly used for removing debris and plaque. It also has some additional functions, like whitening teeth and freshening breath.
   Abrasive, binder, surfactant and humectant are the essential components of toothpaste, among all the other ingredients used. A fluoride containing toothpaste is recommended by the scientific and dental community.

2. **Tooth Powder:** It is a substitute of toothpaste and is available in both fluoride and non-fluoride forms.

3. **Mouthwash:** It is available in a variety of compositions, claiming to kill bacteria forming plaque or bad breath, and freshen up breath on regular use. Basically, they are used after brushing but can also be used prior to brushing.

It is recommended that mouthwash should be used as an aid to brushing rather than a replacement. This is because plaque cannot be easily removed by chemicals alone, and mechanical force required for its removal. Mouthwash or mouth rinse is a product used to enhance oral hygiene, cleanse and freshen up mouth.

Mouthwashes also remove mucus and food particles deeper down in the throat. Alcoholic and strong flavored mouthwashes may cause coughing when used for this purpose.

Examples: Following are the compounds used as dentifrices:

1. Calcium Carbonate,
2. Strontium Chloride,
3. Dibasic Calcium Phosphate,
4. Calcium Phosphate, etc.

Q.4. Write a note on Calcium Carbonate as a dentifrice.

Dentifrices: A dentifrice is a substance used for cleaning the reachable surfaces of the teeth with a toothbrush. The main objective of a dentifrice is to help the toothbrush clean the teeth. Brushing of teeth with or without a dentifrice is beneficial to dental health. A dentifrice is used to maintain good oral hygiene.

Calcium Carbonate ($CaCO_3$): In precipitated calcium carbonate (mol. wt. 100.087) or precipitated chalk, calcium equivalent to or not less than 98% of $CaCO_3$ is detected, when it is dried for 4 hours at 200°C.

Method of Preparation: Calcium carbonate used at industrial level is extracted by mining or quarrying. Calcium carbonate for using in nutraceutical or pharmaceutical industry is extracted from pure quarried source (usually marble).

By calcining crude calcium carbonate, calcium oxide can be prepared. Calcium hydroxide is produced by adding water to the solution and calcium carbonate can be precipitated by passing carbon dioxide through this solution. This calcium carbonate is termed as **precipitated calcium carbonate (PCC).**

$$CaCO_3 \rightarrow CaO + CO_2$$
$$CaO + H_2O \rightarrow Ca(OH)_2$$
$$Ca(OH)_2 + CO_2 \rightarrow CaCO_3 + H_2O$$

Physical Properties: Calcium carbonate is a white fine powder with melting point 825°C.

Chemical Properties:

1. It releases carbon dioxide by reacting with strong acids.

$$CaCO_{3(s)} + 2HCl_{(aq)} \rightarrow CaCl_{2(aq)} + CO_{2(g)} + H_2O_{(l)}$$

2. It releases carbon dioxide and forms calcium oxide (also known as **quicklime**) by heating at 840°C with reaction enthalpy 178 kJ/mole.

$$CaCO_3 \rightarrow CaO + CO_2$$

3. It forms the soluble calcium bicarbonate by reacting with water and carbon dioxide. Erosion of carbonate rocks, formation of caverns andhard water in many regions occurs via this reaction.

$$CaCO_3 + CO_2 + H_2O \rightarrow Ca(HCO_3)_2$$

Medicinal Uses:

1. It is used in most of the toothpastes and toothpowders as a dental cleaning and polishing agent.
2. It is used as an inexpensive dietary calcium supplement or an antacid.
3. It is used for treating hyperphosphatemia in patients with chronic renal failure by acting as a phosphate binder.
4. It is also used as an inert filler for tablets and other pharmaceuticals in

Q.5. Give a detail note on Anticaries Agents. Give preparation and uses of Sodium Fluoride.

Anticaries Agents/Fluorides: When act on carbohydrates, acids are produced which causes dental caries or tooth decay, i.e., decalcification of tooth, along with foul mouth odour.

Classification: Anticaries agents are of two types:

1. Systemic Fluoride
2. Topical Fluoride

1. Systemic Fluorides: Fluorides available in the form of fluorinated water, fluoride drops, and topical fluoride dentifrices are used for preventing tooth decay or dental caries. Tooth decay occurs due to the action of lactic acid which facilitates the formation of plaque on the tooth surface. Flossing and brushing, along with administering fluoride (either, internally or externally) on teeth are the current approaches to prevent dental caries. When hydroxyl in the bones and teeth gets replaced by fluoride in hydroxyapatite, fluoride deposits on bones and teeth. Fluoride inhibits the formation of caries by decreasing the solubility of enamel in acid and bacterial inhibition.

2. Topical Fluorides: These agents are more effective in fluoridated compounds.

Example:

1. **Fluoride Mouthwashes:** They are dispensed in plastic containers and used to inhibit caries. Fluorigard is an **example** of fluoride mouthwash with an aqueous solution of a 0.05% NaF, 15% glycerin, 5% alcohol, and a detergent, a preservative, saccharin, coloring and flavoring agents added as its ingredients.

2. **Fluoride Solutions and Gels:** These are generally formulated with 2% sodium fluoride, 8% stannous fluoride, and acidulated phosphate-fluoride. Fluoride solutions and gels effectively reduces 30-40% dental caries in children. Concentrated fluoride solutions meant for topical use are effective in children with high caries activity because they have both caries arresting and preventive property.

3. **Fluoride Dentifrices:** These agents contain sodium fluoride. Dentifrices currently in use contain sodium mono fluorophosphate, sodium fluoride, or stannous fluoride. Caries is reduced to 25% when these are used regularly. Various dentifrices have been prepared which provide 1000ppm of fluoride. Dentifrices with

0.76% mono fluorophosphate reduce 17-42% dental caries. Sodium fluoride and stannous fluoride are used rarely. Dentifrice with organic amine fluorides are strong plaque-reducers.

4. **Miscellaneous (Listermint with Fluoride):** These are aqueous solutions with 0.02% NaF, 7% glycerine, and alcohol added as ingredients (as in fluorigard). Fluoride is a desensitizing agent and reduces dental hypersensitivity when applied topically. Dental hypersensitivity can also be reduced by using 8% stannous fluoride gels and 33.3% sodium fluoride paste.

Examples:

1. Sodium fluoride,
2. Sodium metaphosphate,
3. Stannous fluoride, and
4. Zinc chloride.

Sodium Fluoride (NaF): Sodium fluoride (mol. wt. 42.0) is a colorless inorganic compound which is a source of the fluoride ion. It is less expensive and hygroscopic than the potassium fluoride.

Methods of Preparation:

1. It can be obtained when sodium hydroxide or sodium carbonate (with equivalent amount of 40% hydrofluoric acid), or hydrogen fluoride is passed into a solution of sodium carbonate.

$$Na_2CO_3 + 2HF \rightarrow 2NaF + H_2O + CO_2$$

2. It can also be prepared by treating mineral cryolite (AlF_3, $3NaF$) with excess of sodium hydroxide. Aluminum fluoride is soluble in the alkali solution and undissolved sodium fluoride is extracted with hot water.

3. Double decomposition of calcium fluoride with sodium carbonate also yields sodium fluoride and insoluble calcium carbonate which is removed by filtration.

$$CaF_2 + Na_2CO_3 \rightarrow 2NaF + CaCO_3\uparrow$$

Physical Properties: Sodium fluoride is a white colored, odorless solid with 993°C melting point.

Chemical Properties:

1. It liberates hydrogen fluoride when treated with concentrated sulphuric acid. This hydrogen fluoride gas attacks silica and silicates.

$$Na_2SiO_3 + 6HF \rightarrow Na_2SiF_6 + 3H_2O$$

2. It is an ionic salt which gives reactions for fluoride and sodium ions. It gives a yellow coloured alizarin-sulphonic acid when reacted with red coloured zirconium-alizarin. A colourless zirconi-fluoride ion is formed during the reaction.

Medicinal Uses:

1. It is used as adjunct to diet and oral hygiene for preventing dental caries.

2. It makes the teeth enamel resistant to acid, promotes re-mineralization It or reduces production of microbial acid.

Q.6. Write about role of Fluoride in the treatment of Dental Caries.

Anticaries Agents/Fluorides: When act on carbohydrates, acids are produced which causes dental caries or tooth decay, i.e., decalcification of tooth, along with foul mouth odour.

Role of Fluoride in the Treatment of Dental Caries: Fluoride is generally added in dentifrices to prevent dental caries. Outstanding results are obtained when trace amount of fluoride salts is applied topically to the teeth.

In human body, fluoride ion is present in trace amount and sufficient quantity is usually obtained from food and water. But places where ground water is lacking in fluoride element, dental problems (like dental caries) are more common and prevalent.

The process of adding fluoride to the municipal water supply is termed as **fluoridation**. This is generally performed to reduce and prevent dental caries. However, slow continued ingestion of fluoride may result in teeth mottling, increased bone density, gastric disturbances, muscular weakness, convulsions, and even heart failure. But, due to its effectiveness in treating dental caries and other types of osteoporosis, fluorides are frequently used in dental practice.

The fluorides can be administered either through oral or topical route. After the internal administration of fluoride salt or solution, it is rapidly absorbed, transported and deposited in the bone or developing teeth. The remaining concentration of fluorides is excreted through kidneys.

The fluoride deposited on the surface of teeth is required to prevent dental carries and is also required to avoid the occurrence of lesions on the teeth surfaces due to action of acids or enzymes. A small quantity of fluoride (1ppm) is usually added in the preparation, whereas more quantity of fluoride (more than 2-3ppm) may cause mottling of teeth enamel and is usually known as **dental fluorosis.**

The fluoridation of public water supply is the most common and efficient means of oral administration. Usually 0.5-1ppm of fluoride salts are added in the water supply. It should be added to drinking water or fruit juice in concentration not more than 1ppm per day. About 2.2mg of sodium fluoride tablets or solution are used per day. Approximately 2% solution of fluoride is applied topically over teeth.

Fluorides either work by **reducing the ability of bacteria to make acids** or by **re-mineralizing the areas of the tooth** that have been attacked by acids from bacteria.

Mechanism of Action: The fluoride ion (F^-) is known to **replace the hydroxyl ion (OH^-)in hydroxyl apatite**, which is the main crystalline structure of enamel. The replaced crystal is known as **fluorapatite** which is more resistant to acids produced by plaque bacteria than the hydroxyl apatite. The absorption of fluoride into enamel can be illustrated through the following chemical reaction:

$$Ca_{10}(PO_4)_6(OH)_2 + 2F^- \rightarrow Ca_{10}(PO_4)_6F_2 + 2(OH)^-$$

Fluoride is an anti-enzyme and generally inhibits the activity of enzymatic acid produced by plaque bacteria. However, the tooth develops and enamelis formed, ingested fluoride gets incorporated into the enamel. In comparison to inner layers, more fluoride is required to develop the outer layer of enamel. The fluoride deposited on the surface enamel layer provides protection against caries.

Examples:

1. Sodium fluoride,
2. Sodium metaphosphate,
3. Stannous fluoride, and
4. Zinc chloride.

Q.7. what are desensitizing agents? Classify desensitizing agents and write a note on Zinc-eugenol Cement.

Desensitizing Agents: Desensitising agents are that relieve painful sensations occurring in exposed dentin and cementum. These agents, however, do not produce immediate relief and should be used for several days or weeks to attain desired results.

First time in the 1920s, aqueous solutions of iodine with silver iodide were reported to be effective for relieving dentinal sensitivity. In the year 1935 **Growman** recommended the standards while selecting a suitable desensitizing agent.

The properties of an **ideal desensitizing agent** are:

1. It should be non-irritating to the pulp.

2. It should be relatively painless on application,

3. Its application should be easy and convenient,

4. Its action should be rapid,

5. Its effects should be permanent and long lasting, and

6. It should not have any decolorizing effects on tooth structure.

Classification: Desensitizing agents can be divided into two types:

1. Chemical Desensitizing agents and

2. Physical Desensitizing agents

Chemical and Physical Agents Used to Treat Dentin Sensitivity

Mode of Action	Agents
Chemical: Anti-inflammatory Protein-precipitating Tubule-occluding	Corticosteroids. Silver nitrate, Zinc chloride, Strontium chloride, Formaldehyde. Calcium hydroxide, Potassium nitrate, Fluorides, Sodium citrate, Iontophoresis with 2% sodium Fluoride, Potassium oxalate.
Physical: Tubule-sealing Physical protection	Composites, Resins, Varnishes, Sealants, Glass ionomer cements, Laser sealing of tubules. Soft tissue grafts.

Zinc-Eugenol Cement: Zinc-eugenol cement or Zinc Oxide Eugenol (ZOE) is formed by combining zinc oxide and eugenol present in clove oil. Zinc eugenol atechelate is formed by an acid-base reaction. Water acts as the catalyst and the metal salts present act as an accelerator in this reaction.

ZOE is used in dentistry when a deeper or decay close to the nerve or pulp chamber occurs. **Acute** or **chronic pulpitis** occurs when the tissue inside the tooth (ie., the pulp) becomes severely inflamed. This results in chronic tooth sensitivity or actual toothache which can be treated only if the nerve (pulp) is removed. This treatment is known as **Root Canal Therapy (RCT)**.

Composition:

1. Zinc oxide (~69.0%),
2. White resin (-29.3%),
3. Zinc acetate (~1.0%),
4. Zinc stearate (~0.7%), and
5. Liquid (eugenol, -85%, olive oil -15%).

Zinc acetate improves strength and zinc stearate acts as an accelerator.

Uses:

1. In dentistry as a filling or cement material,
2. In temporary filling for treating dental caries,
3. In an impression material during construction of complete dentures,
4. In the mucostatic technique of taking impressions, and

5. As an antimicrobial additive in paint.

Q.8. Give Definition of-

1. Cement and Fillers,
2. Oral antiseptics and Astringents
3. Polishing agents/ Abrasive agents

1. Cement and Fillers: Dental cements are mixtures of powder and liquid. These are hard, brittle materials which are either resin cements or acid-base cements. In the latter, the powder is a basic metal oxide or silicate and the liquid is an acid. An acid-base reaction forms a metal salt which acts as the cementing matrix.

Dental cements have a wide range of dental and orthodontic applications, including its use as luting agents, pulp-protecting agents, or cavity-lining materials. They also form an insulating layer under metallic or ceramic restorations. This insulating layer provides protection to the pulp against injury. This helps in sealing or fixing and casting inlays, on lays or any such substance to both dentin and enamel.

The properties **of ideal cement and fillers** are:

1. It should not cause irritation to pulp and gingiva (gums) and should not support the growth of secondary caries.
2. It should form a strong bond between enamel and dentin.
3. It should provide a good marginal sealing, thus, avoiding marginal leakage.
4. It should be resistant to dissolution in saliva or in any oral fluid.

5. It should have good aesthetics, and thermal and chemical resistance.

6. It should be translucent.

2.Oral Antiseptics and Astringents: Certain inorganic substances are used as antiseptics for oral cavity. The antiseptic and/or astringent property of such compounds is utilized to maintain oral hygiene.

Antiseptic agents prevent microbial growth; they are either bacteriostatic or bactericidal. They are used in formulation of oral chemotherapeutic agents as they show very little oral or systemic toxicity, microbial resistance and most of them have broad antimicrobial spectrum. They exhibit either bactericidal activity (killing the microbes) or bacteriostatic activity (affecting the metabolism or reproduction of the microbe). The agent's ability to bind with oral tissues and then be released over a period of time determines the effectiveness of that oral antiseptic agent.

3. Polishing Agents/Abrasive Agents: The major goal of a good dentifrice is to have polishing effect on cleaned teeth by abrasive action. The overall effect is teeth whitening. Besides this, some desensitizing agents are also added in dentifrices for minimizing the teeth sensitivity towards heat and cold. The numbing effect produced by it for short duration is like that of local anesthetics. Astringent type compounds possess this property and thus, are included in dental products. **Examples** of abrasive agent are calcium carbonate, dicalcium phosphate dehydrate, alumina, and silica.

Polishing or abrasive agents are used to remove stained pellicle and plaque from surface of tooth, as well as these agents also to enhance enamel whiteness.

Q.9. Define Mouthwash with different compositions and its types.

Mouthwash: It is available in a variety of compositions, claiming to kill bacteria forming plaque or bad breath, and freshen up breath on regular use. Basically, they are used after brushing but can also be used prior to brushing. It is recommended that mouthwash should be used as an aid to brushing rather than a replacement.

This is because plaque cannot be easily removed by chemicals alone, and mechanical force required for its removal. Mouthwash or mouth rinse is a product used to enhance oral hygiene, cleanse and freshen up mouth.

Mouthwashes also remove mucus and food particles deeper down in the throat. Alcoholic and strong flavored mouthwashes may cause coughing when used for this purpose.

Several mouthwashes with different compositions are available:

i. **Zinc sulphate** is added to provide mild antiseptic and astringent action,

ii. **Zinc chloride** is added to provide deodorant and desensitizing action,

iii. **Potassium permanganate** is added to provide anti-infective and astringent action,

iv. **Sodium bicarbonate** is added to provide antacid property,

v. **Sodium chloride** is added for irrigation, and

vi. **Ammoniacal silver nitrate solution** is added to provide astringent action and to reduce hypersensitivity of teeth and gums.

Following three types of mouthwashes are commonly used:

i. **Plaque Inhibiting:** Used for preventing dental plaque and diseases.

ii. **Anti-gingivitis:** Used for preventing gum diseases.

iii. **Fluoride:** Used for strengthening enamel, preventing cavities, or repairing the existing ones to some extent.

UNIT – 3
GASTROINTESTINAL AGENTS

Q.1. Define gastrointestinal agents? Classify those giving suitable examples.

Gastrointestinal agents: Gastrointestinal agents are used to treating gastrointestinal disorders or diseases. Various organic and inorganic compounds have been classified under the name of gastrointestinal agents that show their relevant actions.

Classification:

1. Inorganic gastrointestinal agents
2. Organic gastrointestinal agents

1. Inorganic gastrointestinal agents:

- ➤ Drugs to neutralize acid for altering gastric pH, **e.g.,** Antacids.
- ➤ Protective for intestinal inflammation, **e.g.,** Charcoal.
- ➤ Adsorbents for intestinal toxins, **e.g.,** Kaolin.
- ➤ Cathartic and Laxatives, **e.g.,** Magnesium sulphate.

2. Inorganic gastrointestinal agents:

- ➤ Drugs for suppressing acid secretion, **e.g.,** Omeprazole

- ➤ Drugs for altering the GI movement, **e.g.,** Cinitapride.
- ➤ Cathartic and Laxatives, **e.g.,** Ispaghula

Q.2 Define acidifiers with examples and give their classifications.

Acidifiers: Drugs that are used to increase metabolic acidosis are known as acidifiers. These agents enhance the acidity of the gastrointestinal tract. Few of these agents are used to increase metabolic acidosis and some of these are used to enhance gastric acid secretion.

Examples of some common acidifiers are:

1. Ammonium chloride,
2. Dilute hydrochloric acid,
3. Phosphoric acid,
4. Fumaric acid, etc.

Classification: The four types of acidifiers are as follows:

1. Gastric Acidifiers
2. Urinary Acidifiers
3. Systemic Acidifiers
4. Acids

1. Gastric Acidifiers: These agents are used to treat patients suffering from achlorhydria or hypochlorhydria. They are helpful to restore the acidity of the stomach temporarily.

Patients suffering from achlorhydria due to chronic alcoholism, tuberculosis, hyperthyroidism, and elderly persons (above 50 years) respond to stimulation of histamine. Therefore, it is possible to treat such patients with histamine phosphate.

In contrast, symptoms of total achlorhydria are observed in suffering from carcinoma of the stomach, chronic gastritis, and gastrectomy. These patients can be treated with hydrochloric acid e some suitable acidifying agent.

Similarly, in pernicious anaemia the deficiency of intrinsic factor is essentially related to the absence of hydrochloric acid. Therefore, dilute hydrochloric acid is generally preferred to counter the effect of achlorhydria.

2. Urinary Acidifiers: These drugs are known to acidify the urine in order to treat certain urinary tract disorders.

3. Systemic Acidifiers: These drugs neutralize the alkaline body fluids (especially blood) in patients suffering from systemic alkalosis.

4. Acids: These are usually used as pharmaceutical aids in the formulations, laboratory quality control, etc.

Q.3. Write the preparation, assay and uses of ammonium chloride.

Ammonium Chloride (NH_4Cl): Ammonium chloride (molecular weight 53.50) is having not less than 99.5% of ammonium chloride which has been calculated with respect to the substance dried for 4 hours over silica gel.

Methods of Preparation:

1. It can be prepared by the reaction of ammonia gas liquors with lime, resulting in the liberation of ammonia which is passed through hydrochloric acid.

2. Ammonium chloride is also formed as the by-product of the Solvay Process. In this process carbon dioxide and ammonia are passed into a cold saturated solution of sodium chloride.

$$CO_2 + 2\ NH_3 + 2\ NaCl + H_2O \rightarrow 2\ NH_4Cl + Na_2CO_3$$

3. On a commercial scale, it can be obtained by the reaction of ammonia gas with hydrochloric acid, followed by the evaporation of the resultant solution to dryness.

$$NH_3 + HCl \rightarrow NH_4Cl$$

The purification of the residue obtained is done by sublimation or crystallization. In the sublimation process, any volatile iron salt is prevented from getting sublimed by mixing salt with 5% calcium phosphate during the process of purification. Generally, the sublimation is performed in cast iron pots which are lined with fire clay having a dome of glass.

Assay: Ammonium chloride is assayed by precipitation titration, using Volhard's method. The steps involved in this method are as follows:

1. 0.2gm of accurately weighed NHCI is dissolved in 40ml of water.

2. The solution is then acidified by adding 3ml of nitric acid.

3. The resultant solution is added with 50ml of N/10 silver nitrate and 5ml of nitrobenzene and is shaken vigorously.

4. A solution of N/10 ammonium thiocyanate is used for titrating excess silver nitrate, using ferric ammonium sulphate (2ml) as an indicator.

$$NH_4Cl + AgNO_3 \rightarrow NH_4NO_3 + AgCl$$
Each ml of 0.IN $AgNO_3$ = 0.005349gm of NH.C1

Now, the assay of ammonium chloride is carried by acid-base titration, which is an inexpensive and simple method (because no silver nitrate is needed).

The steps involved in the assay of ammonium chloride are as follows:

1. Accurately weighed 0.1gm of NH_4Cl is transferred to a conical flask and 50ml of water is added to dissolve it.

2. The solution is then added to 5mlof neutralised formaldehyde solution. This formaldehyde solution may contain little amount of formic acid formed due to atmospheric oxidation; therefore, it should be carefully neutralised with dilute sodium hydroxide solution, using phenolphthalein as an indicator. No excess alkali should be present in this reagent.

3. The resultant solution is kept aside for a couple of minutes and then the liberated hydrochloric acid is titrated with standard sodium hydroxide solution, using some more of phenolphthalein indicator.

1ml of 0.IN sodium hydroxide = 0.005349gm of NH_4C1

4. Ammonium chloride is hydrolysed to produce ammonium hydroxide and hydrogen chloride. The addition of formaldehyde further accelerates this reaction since it fixes ammonia by forming hexamine.

5. The acid is later titrated with alkali without any interruptions. These reactions are illustrated as:

$$NH_4Cl + H_2O \rightarrow NH_4OH + HCl$$
$$4NH_4OH + 6CH_2O \rightarrow C_6H_{12}N_4 + 10H_2O$$
$$HCl + NaOH \rightarrow NaCl + H_2O$$

Properties:

1. Ammonium chloride is a white or colourless crystalline or coarse powder.

2. It is a slightly hygroscopic, odourless inorganic salt with a cooling saline taste.

3. It is freely soluble in water and glycerine, but sparingly soluble in alcohol.

4. A freshly prepared aqueous solution of ammonium chloride is neutral to litmus but rapidly becomes acidic on standing because of hydrolysis.

$$NH_4Cl + 2H_2O \rightarrow NH_4OH + H_2O + Cl^-$$

It is incompatible with the carbonates of alkaline earth metals, lead salts, and with alkalis.

Medicinal Uses:

1. At the same time, also used as an acidifier, as this salt results in increased acidity concentrations of free hydrogen ions.

2. It regulates acid-base equilibrium between the body fluids. Ammonia can be produced by the deamination of amino acids which occurs in the kidney retaining sodium ion.

3. It is used as a diuretic for people with edema or Laennex diseases. A dose of nine grams per day is recommended. Ammonium chloride acts by increasing the renal excretion of chloride.

4. Ammonium chloride, handles an expectorant, helping to irritate the mucosa that is causing the stimulation of the glands of the bronchial mucosa.

5. In the area of pharmacokinetics, ammonium chloride, helps absorb from the GI tract for a period of five to six hours after ingestion.

6. This salt is used for producing dry cells of tin in zinc process and galvanizing processes. In various industries it is used as flux for soldering and metal oxide remover. It is also used in textiles and pottery.

7. Consumption of ammonium chloride should be under medical supervision and with prior registration as it may be harmful for some people, such as those who have been diagnosed with cirrhosis or liver disease.

8. This salt should never be used as treatment of metabolic alkalosis because it can cause a lack of control in renal dysfunction.

Q.4. Write the preparation, properties and uses of Dilute Hydrochloric Acid.

Dilute Hydrochloric Acid (HCl): Dilute hydrochloric acid (molecular weight 36.5) is a solution of hydrogen chloride in water. It is a highly corrosive, strong mineral acid and has extensive industrial use. Naturally, it is present in gastric secretion.

Method of Preparation:

About 9.5-10.5% w/v of HCl is present in dilute hydrochloric acid. It is formed by adding sufficient amount of concentrated hydrochloric acid to water (in the ratio 137: 363). It is stored below 30°C in an airtight container of glass or other inert material.

Properties:

1. It is a clear, colourless, and strongly acidic solution with specific gravity between 1.04-1.05.

2. It can be stored in an airtight container or any inert material below 30°C.

3. It acts as a monoprotic acid and is able to donate one proton per molecule during dissociation and can produce one H^+ ion (a single proton). While in the case of aqueous hydrochloric acid, the H^+ ion combines with one water molecule to form H_3O^+ ion (hydronium ion).

$$HCl + H_2O \rightarrow H_3O^+ + Cl^-$$

Another ion formed in the above reaction is the chloride ion (Cl⁻). Hence, hydrochloric acid can be used in the preparation of salt of chlorides i.e., sodium chloride. The hydrochloric acid is completely ionized in an aqueous solution and acts as a strong acid.

Medicinal Uses:

1. It acts as an acidifying agent.
2. It reacts with organic bases to form hydrochloride salts (soluble in water).
3. It is also used to examine their alkaline properties and to remove the basic drugs. About 25-50ml volume of water can be used further to dilute the hydrochloric acid.
4. It is also used to cure achlorhydria (decreased level of hydrochloric acid in gastric acid) and can also acts as a gastric acidifier.

Q.5. What is an antacid? Give ideal properties and limitation.

Antacids: Compounds used to neutralize the excess amount of acid in the stomach are called antacids. Excess of acid may cause many severe problems like pain, and ulceration, and also inactivate the pepsin (proteolytic enzyme).

The stomach pH ranges from 1 (when empty) to 7 (when food is present). The low acid pH is due to the presence of endogenous hydrochloric acid, which is always present under physiological conditions.

Hyperacidity may lead to heartburn (gastric acid enters into the oesophagus), gastritis (a general inflammation of the gastric mucosa), and peptic ulcer (specific circumscribed erosion).

Ideal Properties:

1. It should be non-absorbable because it may cause systemic alkalosis on getting absorbed systemically
2. It should not cause constipation
3. It should act rapidly for a prolonged time period
4. Its pH should lie within the range of 4-6
5. It should not evolve a large amount of gas on reacting with gastric hydrochloric acid
6. It should inhibit pepsin
7. It should not interfere with food absorption
8. It should be palatable and inexpensive.

Limitations: Long and continuous use of antacid is strictly prohibited. Other limitations of antacids are:

1. Use of antacids is prohibited in patients suffering from renal impairment.
2. Gastric absorption of tetracycline antibiotics is reduced by calcium aluminium, and magnesium antacids.
3. Absorption of digoxin, isoniazid, phenytoin, and warfarin is also reduced in the presence of aluminium hydroxide antacid.
4. Absorption of oral anti-cholinergic agents, phenothiazines and oral iron products is impaired in the presence of antacids.
5. Excretion of acidic drugs (e.g., salicylic acid) is accelerated and urinary excretion of basic drugs (amphetamine) is inhibited in the presence of systemic antacids. Antacids should not be used for a long duration.

Q.6. Define antacid with examples and give their classifications.

Antacids: Compounds used to neutralize the excess amount of acid in the stomach are called antacids. Excess of acid may cause many severe problems like pain, and ulceration, and also inactivate the pepsin (proteolytic enzyme). The stomach pH ranges from 1 (when empty) to 7 (when food is present). The low acid pH is due to the presence of endogenous hydrochloric acid, which is always present under physiological conditions. Hyperacidity may lead to heartburn (gastric acid enters into the oesophagus), gastritis (a general inflammation of the gastric mucosa), and peptic ulcer (specific circumscribed erosion).

Examples of some common antacids:

1. Sodium bicarbonate,
2. Aluminium hydroxide gel,
3. Magnesium hydroxide mixture,
4. Calcium carbonate,
5. Milk of magnesia, etc.

Classification: These are classified in following two types.

1. Systemic Antacids
2. Non-Systemic Antacids

1. Systemic Antacids: These are readily soluble, absorbable, and capable of producing systemic electrolytic alterations and alkalosis. **Example** Sodium bicarbonate.

2.Non-Systemic Antacids: These are not absorbed to a significant extent and thus do not exert a systemic effect. **Examples** Aluminium salts, Magnesium salts, Calcium carbonate, and Sodium carboxyethyl cellulose.

Q.7. Write the preparation, assay and uses of Sodium Bicarbonate.

Sodium Bicarbonate (Baking Soda, NaHCO$_3$): Sodium bicarbonate (molecular weight 84.01) is not having less than 99% and not more than 101% of sodium bicarbonate.

Methods of Preparation:

1. It can be prepared by passing strong brine having high contents of ammonia through a carbonating tower, where the saturation takes place under pressure with dioxide. After that, the ammonia is treated with carbon dioxide to form ammonia bicarbonate that reacts with sodium chloride to give sodium bicarbonate (as precipitate). By filtration, it can be separated out.

2. It can also be prepared by treating sodium carbonate crystals with an aqueous solution such as water. After that, a sufficient amount of carbon dioxide is passed through it to saturation.

Assay: 1gm of sodium bicarbonate is weighed accurately and dissolved. The resultant mixture is titrated with 0.5N H$_2$SO$_4$ using methyl water Orange as an indicator.

Each ml of 0.5N H$_2$SO$_4$ = 0.042gm of NaHCO$_3$

Properties:

Sodium bicarbonate is an odourless, white crystalline powder with slightly alkaline taste. It is stable only in dry air, and is sparingly soluble in water and insoluble in organic solvent (e.g., alcohol, ether, etc.). Chemically, it can be converted into sodium sesquicarbonate (Na2CO3.NaHCO3.2H$_2$O) at 100°C. It is an alkaline solution and produces effervescence by reacting with acids.

Medicinal Uses:

1. In pharmaceutical preparations, sodium bicarbonate is used as acid neutralizing agent.
2. It is used to combat systemic acidosis, and acts as an antacid.
3. It is used in the preparation of buffer solutions (NaHCO3 + H$_2$CO3).
4. Its aqueous solutions are used as local applicants for burns, and insect bites. etc. It is also a constituent of an effervescent mixture.
5. It can be used as a local applicant for burns, insect bites, etc. in the form of aqueous solutions.

Q.8. Write the preparation, properties and uses of Aluminium hydroxide gel.

Aluminium Hydroxide Gel [Amphojel, Al(OH)$_3$]: Aluminium hydroxide is a non-systemic, weak antacid. Preparations of aluminium hydroxide gel (molecular weight 78) should not have less than 3.5% and not more than 4.4% w/w of aluminium oxide (Al$_2$O$_3$).

Methods of Preparation:

1. Aluminium hydroxide is precipitated in a gelatinous form by adding ammonia to a solution of aluminium salt. Potash alum ($K_2SO_4.Al_2(SO_4)_3.18H_2O$) may be used as a source of aluminium salt. On heating the mixture, the hydroxide becomes amorphous. This amorphous mixture is filtered, washed with hot water, and dried.

$$Al^{3+}+3OH^- \rightarrow Al(OH)_3\downarrow$$

2. It can be formed by treating an aluminium salt (e.g., aluminium chloride or sulphate) with ammonium hydroxide.

$$AlCl_3+3NH_4OH \rightarrow Al(OH)_3+3NH_4Cl$$

Properties:

1. Aluminium hydroxide is a white coloured gel
2. It is soluble in acids and alkalis
3. Melting point of aluminium hydroxide is 300°C.

Chemical reactions:

1. Aluminium hydroxide gel is an amphoteric compound and acts as ideal buffer at a pH range of 3-5.

$$\textbf{Base + Acid} \leftrightarrow \textbf{Conjugate acid conjugate base}$$

2. It yields aluminium chloride when treated with hydrochloric acid.

$$Al(OH)_3 +3HCl \rightarrow AlCl_3+3H_2O$$

3. It gets converted to aluminium oxide on heating.

$$2Al(OH)_3 + \rightarrow Al_2O_3 + 3H_2O$$

4. It acts as an acid in the presence of an alkali.

$$Al(OH)_3 \leftrightarrow 3H^+ + AlO_3^{3-}$$

5. It acts as weak in the presence of an acid.

$$Al(OH)_3 \leftrightarrow Al^{3+} + OH^-$$

Medicinal Uses:

1. To treat peptic ulcer, gastritis, peptic esophagitis, gastric hyperactivity, and hiatal hernia.

2. To protect the skin and used as a mild astringent.

3. To adsorb pepsin due to adsorbent properties.

Q.9. Write the preparation, properties and uses of Magnesium hydroxide mixture.

Magnesium Hydroxide Mixture [Milk of Magnesia, $Mg(OH)_2$]: Magnesium hydroxide (molecular weight 58.3197) or milk of magnesia contains not less than 95% and not more than 100.5% of $Mg(OH)_2$.

Method of Preparation: Magnesium hydroxide is obtained in the form of smooth cream on reaction of sodium hydroxide with magnesium sulphate. This smooth, creamy product is diluted with water form suspension which is poured into magnesium sulphate solution by constant stirring. A precipitate is obtained which is allowed to settle and the upper clear liquid is removed by decantation.

The residue is transferred on a calico filter, washed with water to remove sulphate ions, and then desired volume is obtained by mixing the precipitate with sufficient water.

$$MgO + 3H_2O \rightarrow Mg(OH)_2$$
$$MgSO_4 + 2NaOH \rightarrow Mg(OH)_2 + Na_2SO_4$$

If magnesium sulphate is mixed with sodium hydroxide, a gelatinous translucent precipitate of magnesium hydroxide is obtained. If magnesium oxide is used along with sodium hydroxide, a white and creamy suspension is formed.

Properties:

1. Magnesium hydroxide is a white coloured, opaque, and more or less viscous suspension.
2. When it is left undisturbed, water separates from it in different proportions.
3. At pH 10, magnesium hydroxide is alkaline to litmus solution and absorbs carbon dioxide from air.

Medicinal Use:

1. Magnesium hydroxide is a non-systemic gastric antacid and mild cathartic.
2. On continuous or prolonged use, kidney stones may develop.

Q.10. Write a note on combination of antacids.

Combinations of Antacids: These combinations are used to maintain the laxative effect of magnesium and the constipated effect of calcium and aluminium. Due to gaseous properties, trimethicone (as deforming agent) has been additionally mixed with some antacids.

Example: for Reflux oesophagitis, Alginic acid (hydrophilic colloidal carbohydrate acid obtained from seaweed) has been added to it.

It is given 1-2 hours after taking a meal and at bedtime. These drugs are administered in the following conditions:

1. In peptic ulcer,
2. In hyperacidity,
3. Gastritis,
4. Heartburn of pregnancy,
5. Reflux oesophagitis, and
6. Flatulent dyspepsia.

It is not possible to fulfil all the criteria for an ideal antacid; many products are composed of mixtures of antacids that are commonly available in the market. Many of these combination products have a laxative effect of magnesium and a constipated effect of calcium. There are also some products which are made up of combination of an antacid and show the rapid onset of action, while other has a longer duration of action

Commercially available combinations of antacid preparations are given below:

1. Aluminium Hydroxide Gel – Magnesium Trisilicate Combination
2. Magaldrate

3. Calcium Carbonate containing Antacid Mixtures

4. Alginic Acid Sodium Bicarbonate – containing Antacid Mixtures

1. Aluminium Hydroxide Gel-Magnesium Trisilicate Combination: It is one of the most common combinations available. It shows laxative protective, and constipated properties.

2. Magaldrate: It is made up of two chemical constituents, i.e., magnesium hydroxide and aluminium hydroxide. It comprises 2 39% of magnesium oxide and about 17-25% of aluminium oxide in the given preparation. It is generally white in colour, odourless crystalline powder which is insoluble in water and any other solve like alcohol. However, it is soluble in the mineral acids (in the form of dilute solutions).

3. Calcium Carbonate containing Antacid Mixtures: Calcium carbonate with a mixture of antacid like aluminium hydroxide gel yields those products which show the prolonged action with a rapid onset (e.g., calcium carbonate, magnesium containing antacid, and aluminium hydroxide gel).

4. Alginic Acid Sodium Bicarbonate-containing Antacid Mixtures: The alginic acid is treated with sodium bicarbonate to produce sodium alginate with carbon dioxide. In gastric acid, alginic acid is precipitated in the presence of light and a type of viscous gel floats on the top of G.I.T.

Q.11. What are cathartics? Classify cathartics giving examples and discuss preparation identification and uses of following:

(a) Magnesium sulphate
(b) Sodium orthophosphate.

Cathartics: Cathartics are therapeutic agents which facilitate defecation. **Purgatives** are similar agents but their nature of action is comparatively milder than cathartics, while laxatives are milder forms of purgatives. They may exert similar therapeutic effects but their nature and mechanism of action are different.

Generally, peristaltic movement is responsible for defecation under normal conditions. The peristaltic waves produced by the stimulation of the muscular layer stimulate the bowel to relieve its contents.

In a healthy person, this peristaltic motion usually occurs around three to four times in a day. In most of the cases, constipation results due to continued ignoring the urge to defecate either voluntary or due to psychological reasons.

Constipation may also occur due to weak intestine, intestinal spasms, and injury. use of certain drugs, diet, etc. The faecal material becomes dry and hard in constipation. Laxatives or purgatives (lubricants) are used in the treatment of constipation since they facilitate the emptying of the bowels.

Classification: On the basis of their mechanism of action cathartics or purgatives can be classified as follows:

1. Stimulants

2. Bulk Purgatives

3. Lubricants

4. Saline Cathartics

1. Stimulants: These drugs or chemicals initiate peristaltic movement by local irritation of intestinal tract. They are termed as stimulants because they act directly on intestine to stimulate peristalsis. Examples of drugs of this class are senna, rhubarb, cascara, podophyllum, castor oil, aloe vera, etc.

2. Bulk Purgatives: These agents act by increasing the bulk of intestinal contents. These are cellulose or non-digestible materials that swell considerably when wet and because of increased bulk they stimulate the peristaltic movement. Examples of drugs of this class are methylcellulose, sodium CMC, gum, ispagol, etc.

3. Lubricants: The intestinal contents absorb water from the body and become hard in constipation, therefore the patient experiences difficulty in emptying bowels. Liquid paraffin, glycerine, mineral oils are few substances that act as lubricants and facilitate emptying of the bowels.

4. Saline Cathartics: They absorb large quantity of water to increase the osmotic load of intestine and thus stimulate peristalsis. Poorly absorbable cations (e.g., calcium, magnesium) and anions (e.g., phosphate, sulphate, tartrate) cause this effect. Generally, saline cathartics are water soluble inorganic chemicals and are taken with plenty of water. They restrict excessive fluid loss from the body and reduce nausea and vomiting.

Example:

1. Magnesium sulphate,
2. Sodium orthophosphate,
3. Kaolin,
4. Bentonite,
5. Sodium phosphate, etc.

(a) Magnesium Sulphate (Epsom Salt, Bitter Salt, $MgSO_4.7H_2O$):

Magnesium sulphate (molecular weight 246.47) is quite abundant in nature in the form of kieserite $MgSO_4.H_2O(MgSO_4.7H_2O)$. A large amount of magnesium sulphate is found in seawater. Magnesium sulphate should not have less than 99.0% of $MgSO_4$.

Methods of Preparation:

1. In laboratory, magnesium sulphate is prepared by neutralisation reaction between hot dilute sulphuric acid with magnesium, or its oxide or carbonate. The solution is filtered, concentrated, and crystallised.
2. On a commercial scale, it is manufactured by the reaction of sulphuric acid with magnesite or with powdered and calcined dolomite Magnesium sulphate so formed dissolves in the solution and a sparingly soluble calcium sulphate is deposited. The liquid is filtered concentrated, and crystallised.

$$MgCO_3.CaCO_3 + 2H_2SO_4 + MgSO_4 + CaSO_4 + 2CO_2 + 2H_2O$$

3. Magnesium sulphate is also prepared from the native sulphate (kieserite), $MgSO_4.H_2O$ by dissolving in hot water. When the solution is cooled, rhombic crystals of heptahydrate are deposited.

Properties:

1. Magnesium sulphate is a white crystalline solid and is anhydrous in nature.
2. It is slightly soluble in alcohol and glycerol.

Chemical reactions:

1. It forms double salt on reacting with ammonium or magnesium hydroxide and with disodium hydrogen phosphate, in the presence of ammonium chloride.

$$MgSO_4 + Na_2HPO_4 + NH_4OH \rightarrow MgNH_4PO_4 + Na_2SO_4 + H_2O$$

2. On heating, it decomposes and sulphur trioxide is evolved.

$$MgSO_4 \rightarrow MgO + SO_3$$

Medicinal Uses:

1. Magnesium sulphate is widely used in medicine as a purgative (orally at a dose of 15-30gm).
2. Subcutaneously, it is used as a spasmolytic agent in hypertension in the form of a 25% solution.
3. Intramuscularly, it is used as a putrefacient in doses of 10-20ml of a 25% solution.
4. It is used as an anti-convulsive agent.

5. Orally, it is used as a biogenic agent in the form of a 20-25% solution.

6. Parentally, it is used as a tranquilizing agent which acts on the central nervous system.

(b) Sodium Orthophosphate $(Na_2HPO_4.12H_2O)$: Sodium orthophosphate (molecular weight 358.14) is a disodium hydrogen orthophosphate or sodium phosphate. It should not have more than 101.0% and less than 98.5% of Na_2HPO_4

Methods of Preparation:

1. It can be prepared by treating sodium carbonate with a hot solution of phosphoric acid. Since it affects the third hydrogen of phosphoric acid, it leads to the formation of disodium hydrogen phosphate. The solution is neutralized concentrated, and the crystals are separated, centrifuged, washed, and dried.

$$H_3PO_4 + Na_2CO_3 \rightarrow Na_2HPO_4 + H_2O + CO_2$$

2. It can also be prepared from calcium phosphate in appropriate concentration with acid which yields monobasic calcium phosphate and calcium sulphate. Finally, the former is precipitated out while the other substances remain in the solution.

$$Ca_3(PO_4)_2 + 2H_2SO_4 \rightarrow Ca(H_2PO_4)_2 + 2CaSO_4 \downarrow$$

The above mixture after the addition of boiling water is filtered. Now, the filtrate is treated with sodium carbonate when dibasic calcium phosphate gets deposited leaving sodium phosphate (disodium hydrogen phosphate) in solution. The reaction may be put as follows:

$$Ca(H_2PO_4)_2 + Na_2CO_3 \rightarrow CaHPO_4 + Na_2HPO_4 + CO_2 + H_2O$$

The remaining solution is then filtered. The crystals of sodium phosphate are obtained while concentrating the solution.

Properties:

1. It is generally found in the form of colourless transparent crystals of saline taste.
2. It is odourless and in air it shows efflorescent property.
3. It is very soluble in water and insoluble in alcohol.
4. It is converted to sodium pyrophosphate at an optimum temperature of 300°C.

Medicinal Uses: It is used as a saline laxative, buffering agent, or a cathartic agent.

Q.12. Write the preparation, properties and uses of Kaolin.

Kaolin ($Al_2O_3.2SiO_2.2H_2O$): Kaolin (molecular weight 258.09) is a natural, purified, hydrated aluminium silicate of varying composition.

It is also known as China clay and is of two types:

1. Heavy kaolin
2. Light kaolin

1. Heavy kaolin:

➤ It is a purified natural form of varying composition.

- The flat particles of diameter of about 20μm are generally found irregularly arranged.
- It usually exists as a fine white or greyish-white earthy mass or powder. Practically, it is insoluble in water and organic solvents (e.g., ether, benzene, alcohol, etc.).
- A plastic-like form of kaolin is less sticky with water.
- Kaolin c down and leaves a clear supernatant liquid when the suspension is kept aside for some time.
- It polarises plane light

2. Light Kaolin:

- It is a natural form of kaolin which is purified by elutriation followed by drying.
- It contains a suitable dispersing a comprises of small (less than 2um in diameter) particles of different shapes and sizes.
- They do not have light polarising property.
- It is a white, light, odourless, and unctuous (free from gritty particles powder.
- It is generally insoluble in water and mineral acids.
- It exists a sticky mass with water.
- Its aqueous suspension is turbid permanently and only small quantity of kaolin is deposited.
- Natural light kaolin (or light kaolin) does not contain any dispersing agent.

Method of Preparation: Kaolin is obtained from the breakdown of feldspar from granite rocks. It obtained after the rock is mined, excavated, and its impurities are washed off with water and then it is powdered. The rock is elutriated with water to separate large-sized particles. The turbid liquid is permitted to settle down, Finally, fractions of heavy kaolin (comprising large particles) and colloidal kaolin (comprising small particles) are separated and dried.

Kaolin meant for pharmaceutical applications is usually purified by treating it with either hydrochloric or sulphuric acid, or both, and then washed thoroughly with water.

Properties:

1. Kaolin is a white coloured, plastic-like substance with an earthy or clay-like taste.
2. Colour of kaolin may be tinted grey, yellow brown, blue or red due to the presence of various impurities.
3. It is soapy and unctuous touch but its surface becomes highly polished rubbing.
4. In the presence of moisture, it appears dark coloured and gives out a clay-like odour.
5. Its fusion point lies between 1700-1800°C.
6. It loses water on heating.
7. It remains unaffected by dilute hydrochloric or nitric acid.
8. Prolonged boiling or exposure to concentrated sulphuric acid may decompose kaolin.
9. In case it is initially heated to white heat, it becomes more resistant to acids.

Medicinal uses:

1. It is used in the treatment of dysentery, symptomatic treatment of colitis, and in cholera.

2. It finds use in the treatment of alkaloidal and food poisoning, as it can readily absorb poisons.

3. It can be used in the preparation of topical agents such as cosmetic preparations, dusting powder, etc.

4. It is also used in the preparation of kaolin poultice employed externally

Q.13. Write the preparation, properties and uses of Bentonite.

Bentonite ($Al_2O_3.4SiO_2.H_2O$): Bentonite (molecular weight of is 549.07) is also known as wilkinite. It is a colloidal, hydrated aluminium silicate comprising of montmorillonite ($Al_2O_3.4SiO_2.H_2O$). Elements like calcium, magnesium. natural. and iron may also be present.

The amount of water in bentonite depends on the extraction method to which the natural substances are subjected. Most commonly found clay bentonite comprises of about 90% montmorillonite ($Al_2Si_4O_{10}(OH)_2.nH_2O$), feldspar ($K_2O.Al_2O_3.6SiO_2$), aluminosilicate containing SiO_2, Al_2O_3, Fe_2O_3, CaO, MgO, and some Na and K salts.

Method of Preparation:

Crude bentonite is reduced to fine particles of small sizes and purified to remove impurities like quartz, muscovite, illite, feldspar, and iron oxide.

These impurities are removed by adding its aqueous solution into a very dilute aqueous solution of an official grade of sodium hexa meta phosphate.

The mixture is allowed to remain undisturbed till all mineral impurities are precipitated. Either filtration or centrifugation techniques are used to separate the purified suspended bentonite from the supernatant liquid.

Properties:

1. Bentonite is an odourless, pale buff, cream-coloured, or greyish-white powder with a yellowish tint.
2. It is free of gritty particles and its taste is slightly earthy.
3. It is usually insoluble in but into a homogeneous mass, it may swell about 12 times the volume of the dry powder.
4. It is insoluble in and does not swell in organic solvents.
5. The pH of 5% suspension of purified bentonite usually lies in the range of about 9.0-10.0.
6. It is mostly stored in tightly closed containers.

Medicinal Uses:

1. Bentonite is a popular pharmaceutical additive and is commonly used as a protective colloid to stabilise emulsions.
2. It is used to suspend different types of insoluble powders.
3. It can also be used as an emulsifier for oil in water emulsions.
4. It is normally used as a base in-various pharmaceutical preparations like plasters and ointments.

5. It is a constituent of calamine lotion I.P. which protects the skin from dust and harmful sun rays.

Q.14. What are antimicrobials? Classify them and give examples?

Antimicrobials: Antimicrobials are agents that either kill or inhibit the growth of microorganisms (bacteria, fungi, or protozoans). These agents are either microbicidal (kill microbes) or micro biostatic (prevent the growth of microbes) in nature. Antimicrobial substances like disinfectants are generally used to clean non-living objects.

Classification: These are chemical preparations used to reduce or prevent microbial infections.

Depending on the mechanism of action they may be of the following types:

1. Antiseptics
2. Disinfectants
3. Germicides
4. Bacteriostatic agents
5. Sanitizers

1. Antiseptics:

➢ These substances are used to inhibit the microbial growth and are specifically applied on living tissues.

➢ Antiseptic agents are used to treat sepsis, putrefaction, or decay of the damaged or exposed tissues.

- They act either by inhibiting multiplication and metabolic activities or microorganisms, or by killing the pathogenic microbes.
- An ideal antiseptic agent should be effective against bacteria, spores, fungi, viruses, or any other infective agent without harming any body tissues of host.
- They must be safe to be applied on almost all body tissues and can be used in the preparation of mouthwashes, soaps, deodorants, throat and nasal sprays, and vaginal douches.
- Generally, antiseptics are protein denaturants and act on bacterial enzymes. Therefore, their activity decreases in serum, blood, or pus.

2. Disinfectants:

- These substances kill the pathogenic microorganisms to prevent infection.
- Disinfectants are usually applied to non-living objects.
- These are frequently used to maintain hygienic conditions in home and hospitals.
- They are bactericidal in nature and cause irreversible toxic effects.
- Disinfection can also be achieved through heat, irradiation, or chemicals.
- Their microbicidal action is non-selective in nature, and therefore they also destroy non-pathogenic microbes.

> All disinfectant solutions undergo degradation, if stored for prolonged time period or at elevated temperature.
> Few chemical disinfectants are known to cause irritation or corrosion to the skin or tissues.

3. Germicides:

> These are substances which kill microorganisms.
> More precise terms like bactericide (against bacteria), fungicide (against fungi), virucide (against virus), etc., generally signify microbes against which they are used or effective.

4. Bacteriostatic Agents:

> These are used to inhibit bacterial growth.
> These drugs or agents do not kill but hamper bacterial growth.

5. Sanitizers:

> These are disinfectants that are used to maintain general public health standards.
> These are used to clean or wash away the organic matter (e.g., saliva, mucous, etc.).
> Germicidal agents are anti-infective agents that are used to kill the microorganisms.
> Their germicidal activity increases with their concentration, but this concentration should not cause any local cellular damage.

> Likewise, if applied topically, they should not cause any systemic toxicity.

Examples:

1. Potassium permanganate,
2. Boric acid,
3. Hydrogen peroxide,
4. Chlorinated lime,
5. Iodine preparations, etc.

Q.15. Define antimicrobial agents with their mechanism and examples.

Antimicrobials: Antimicrobials are agents that either kill or inhibit the growth of microorganisms (bacteria, fungi, or protozoans). These agents are either microbicidal (kill microbes) or micro biostatic (prevent the growth of microbes) in nature. Antimicrobial substances like disinfectants are generally used to clean non-living objects.

Mechanism: The mechanism involved in the antimicrobial action of these agents generally range from a mild astringent to powerful oxidative property. Inorganic compounds are very rarely used as anti-infectives in the treatment of systemic infections. Thus, they are not used internally like other antibiotics or sulphonamides, except in a few cases. If applied topically (dermatological, oral, ear, ophthalmic, etc.) they should be used carefully.

Following three mechanisms are generally employed to exhibit antimicrobial action of inorganic compounds:

1. **Oxidation:** Different compounds belonging to the category of peroxides of peroxyacids, oxygen liberating like permanganate and certain oxo-halogen anions exhibit this mechanism. These agents oxidise the active functional groups present in proteins or enzymes important for the growth and survival of microbes. It results to alteration in configuration of bacterial protein and hence affects their functions.

   Example: A free sulfhydryl group is necessary for activity of a variety of proteins and enzymes. However, this free nature of sulfhydryl group is destroyed through oxidation and results in the formation of a disulphide (disulphide) bond.

2. **Halogenation:** Compounds liberating chlorine and hypochlorite or iodine act by this mechanism. These agents commonly act on peptide linkage and affect its capabilities and properties. A damage to a functional group present in protein results in microbial death.

   Enzymes are proteinaceous compounds and a protein molecule is composed of a long chain of amino acids joined by a peptide (-CONH) linkage. Hypohalite

   Example: Hypochlorite (OC halogenate (chlorinate) peptide linkage, thus antiseptics having hypohalite (hypochlorite) functional groups act as antimicrobial a by chlorinating the peptide linkages in protein molecule.

   The hydrogen-bonding responsible for proper orientation of the protein molecule is altered due to the substitution of chlorine atom on the nitrogen of peptide linkage. Thus, proper functions of the protein are not carried out.

3. **Protein Precipitation:** Most of the metal ions act by protein binding or protein precipitation. The polar group of protein (that acts as ligands) and metal ions (that act as Lewis acid) determines the nature of interaction with protein. However, the resultant complex may be chelating that may inactivate the protein.

This action is usually non-specific since protein precipitants are unable to differentiate between protein of microbe and that of the host. Germicidal action is only attained at such ionic concentration that largely restricts the reaction to the parasite cell. Depending concentration and extent of reaction, actions like astringent, irritant, corrosive, or even caustic action may be seen on the host.

Examples:

6. Potassium permanganate,
7. Boric acid,
8. Hydrogen peroxide,
9. Chlorinated lime,
10. Iodine preparations, etc.

Q.16. Write the preparation, properties and uses of Potassium permanganate.

Potassium Permanganate ($KMnO_4$): Potassium permanganate (molecular weight 158), formerly known as permanganate of potash or **Condy's crystals** is the inorganic, water- soluble chemical compound which consists of equal moles of potassium (K) and permanganate [MnO_4^-, officially called manganate (VII)] ions. This salt is a strong oxidising agent.

Methods of Preparation:

1. It can be prepared by mixing KOH solution, powdered manganese oxide and potassium chlorate. The resultant mixture is boiled and evaporated. The residue obtained is heated in iron pans till it forms a paste of desired consistency.

$$KOH + 3MnO_2 + KClO_3 \rightarrow KMnO_4 + KCl + 3H_2O$$

2. It can be prepared by heating potassium hydroxide and manganese dioxide together in the presence of air or potassium nitrate/potassium chlorate (oxidising agent).

$$2KOH + MnO_2 \rightarrow KMnO_4 + 3H_2O$$

The greenish potassium permanganate formed is treated with$Cl_2/CO_2/H_2O$:

$$3K_2MnO_4 + 2CO_2 \rightarrow 2KMnO_4 + MnO_2 + 2K_2CO_3$$
$$2K_2MnO_4 + Cl_2 \rightarrow 2KMnO_4 + 2KCl$$
$$2K_2MnO_4 + 2H_2O \; 2KMnO_4 + 2KOH + H_2$$

The solutions obtained above are filtered to separate the potassium manganate precipitate. The filtrate is concentrated and potassium permanganate crystals are obtained when the filtrate is cooled.

Properties:

1. Potassium permanganate is found in the form of dark purple coloured monoclinic prism.
2. It is odourless and almost opaque and has a blue metallic lustre.
3. It is soluble in 15 parts of water and 3.5 parts of boiling water.
4. Solution of $KMnO_4$ is sweet and tastes like astringent.
5. On heating at 240°C it disintegrates and deteriorates.
6. It is a powerful oxidising agent

Chemical reaction:

1. On passing HS gas through acidified (with HCl) potassium permanganate solution, the violet colour disappears and sulphur gets precipitated.

   $$2KMnO_4 + 6HCl + 5H_2S \rightarrow 2MnCl_2 + 2KCl + 5S \downarrow + 8H_2O$$

2. On adding a solution of hydrogen peroxide (H_2O_2) potassium permanganate solution, the colour of $KMnO_4$ solution disappears.

   $$2KMnO_4 + 3H_2SO_4 + 5H_2O_2 \rightarrow K_2SO_4 + 2MnSO_4 + 8H_2O + 5O_2$$

3. Chlorine gas is produced on adding hydrochloric acid to a potassium permanganate solution.

   $$2KMnO_4 + 16HCl \rightarrow 2KCl + 2MnCl_2 + 8H_2O + 5Cl_2 \uparrow$$

4. An alkaline or neutral solution of potassium permanganate iodide to iodate.

   $$2KMnO_4 + H_2O + KI \rightarrow 2MnO_2 + 2KOH + KIO_3$$

5. In acidic medium, iodine is liberated from iodides.

$$2KMnO_4 + 10KI + 8H_2SO_4 \rightarrow 6K_2SO_4 + 2MnSO_4 + 5I_2$$
$$+8H_2O$$

6. Ferrous salts get oxidised to ferric salts in an acidic solution.

$$2KMnO_4 + 10FeSO_4 + 8H_2SO_4 \rightarrow K_2SO_4 + 2MnSO_4 +$$
$$Fe_2(SO_4)_3 + 8H_2O$$

Medicinal Uses:

1. Potassium permanganate is used as an antiseptic in mouth washes.
2. It is used in the treatment of urethritis.
3. It oxidises proteins and other bio-organic substances due to its oxidising properties.
4. Its solution destroys the effect of a poison and prevents its absorption.
5. It is used as a disinfectant and deodorant.
6. It is an astringent, anti-infective, and a bactericidal.
7. Its solution is used as wet dressings to clean ulcers or abscesses, and in baths in conditions of eczema and acute dermatoses.
8. Its solution is also used in bromhidrosis (evil smelling perspiration), mycotic infections (athlete's foot, poison ivy dermatitis), and as a stomach wash-out for treating morphine, opium, and strychnine poisoning.

Q.17. Write the preparation, properties and uses of Boric acid.

Boric Acid (H_3BO_3): Boric acid (molecular weight 61.83) occurs naturally as a **sassolite** mineral. It contains 99.5 to 100.5% of HBO, which has been calculated with reference to the dried substance.

Methods of Preparation:

1. **By Decomposition of Borax:** Hot aqueous solution of borax is mixed with a mixture of concentrated sulphuric acid, followed by addition of water. The hot solution is filtered and cooled resulting in the crystallization of boric acid which is separated by filtration.

$$Na_2B_4O_7 + H_2SO_4 + 5H_2O \rightarrow Na_2SO_4 + 4H_3BO_3$$

2. **From Colemanite:** Sulphur dioxide is passed through colemanite suspended in water and the crystals of boric acid forms on cooling.

$$Ca_2B_6O_{11} + 4SO_2 + 11H_2O \rightarrow 2Ca(HSO_3)_2 + 6H_3BO_3$$

Physical Properties:

1. Boric acid is a weak acid which turns litmus paper slightly red.
2. On treating with boric acid, colour of turmeric paper changes to brown which when dipped in sodium hydroxide solution turns blackish.
3. Ethyl alcohol and boric acid mixture burns with a green flame due to the formation of ethyl borate.
4. Boric acid reacts with equimolar amount of glycerine at 140-150°C to produce boroglycerin glycerite ($C_3H_5BO_3$) which is used as a suppository base.

Chemical Properties:

1. Action of heat on boric acid:

1. At100°C, it loses one molecule of water to produce meta boric acid

$$H_3BO_3 \rightarrow HBO_2 + H_2O$$

2. At 160°C, it produces tetra boric acid

$$4H_3BO_3 \rightarrow 5H_2O + H_2B_4O_7$$

3. On heating at high temperature, it forms a glassy mass of boron trioxide

$$4H_3BO_3 \rightarrow 5H_2O + H_2B_4O_7$$

Medicinal Uses:

1. It is used in eyewash and mouthwash in the form of solutions at a concentration of 2.5-4.5%.
2. It is used as an emollient antiseptic ointment for treating diaper rash.
3. It is also used as a dusting powder.
4. It prevents discolouration of physostigmine solutions.
5. It possesses weak bacteriostatic, fungistatic, astringent, and antiseptic properties.
6. It is used as a buffer and as an antimicrobial in eye drops.

Q.18. Write the preparation, assay and uses of Hydrogen peroxide and Chlorinated lime.

Hydrogen Peroxide (H_2O_2):

- Hydrogen peroxide (molecular weight 34) is the simplest stable peroxide (contain oxygen-oxygen single bond).
- It is a weak acid with a powerful bleaching action.
- It is a strong oxidising agent and with highly reactive Oxygen species.
- Hydrogen peroxide is a by-product of oxygen metabolism; thus, it is synthesised naturally in organisms.
- Peroxidases enzymes, present in almost all living cells, decompose low concentrations of hydrogen peroxide harmlessly and catalytically to water and oxygen.

Methods of preparation:

1. **Electrolysis:** In this method, hydrogen peroxide is prepared by the Methods of Preparation electrolysis of 50% ice-cold H2SO4. Electrolysis results in the formation of per disulphuric acid which is distilled under reduced pressure to give 30% H_2O_2. The distillate with H_2O_2 is analysed and is adjusted to get the desired strength.

$$2H_2SO_4 \rightarrow 2HSO_4 + 2H^-$$
$$\text{At cathode } 2H^+ + 2e^- \rightarrow H_2 \uparrow$$
$$\text{At anode } 2HSO_4 + 2e^- \rightarrow H_2S_2O_8$$
$$H_2S_2O_8 + 2H_2O \rightarrow 2H_2SO_4 + H_2O_2$$

2. Decomposition of barium peroxide, with phosphoric acid or passage of carbon dioxide through a suspension of barium peroxide in water gives hydrogen peroxide.

$$3BaO_2 + 2H_3PO_4 \rightarrow Ba_3(PO_4)_2 + 3H_2O_2$$
$$BaO_2 + H_2O + CO_3 \rightarrow H_2O_2 + BaCO_2$$

3. A thick paste of barium peroxide is added in ice-cold water. This mixture is added to a calculated volume of ice-cold dilute sulphuric acid. The solution is filtered and the insoluble sulphate is separated.

$$BaO_2 + H_2SO_4 \rightarrow BaSO_4\downarrow + H_2O_2$$

Assay: Both hydrogen peroxide and acidified potassium permanganate are oxidizing agents, which reduce each other and liberate gaseous oxygen. KMnO4 solution is reduced and discoloured by hydrogen peroxide. An extra drop of KMnO4 produces pink colour at the endpoint. Potassium permanganate itself acts as an indicator.

The permanganate method is used to assay hydrogen peroxide. This method comprises of the following steps:

1. About 10ml of the sample is diluted with 250ml of purified water in a volumetric flask.
2. 10ml of SN sulphuric acid is added to the 25ml of above-mentioned solution
3. The resultant solution is titrated with 0.1N potassium permanganates olution, until a faint pink colour is obtained.

Each ml of 0.1N KMnO$_4$ = 0.001701gm of H$_2$O$_2$

$$2KMnO_4 + 3H_3SO_4 + 5H_2O_2 \rightarrow K_2SO_4 + 8H_2O + 5O_2 + 2MnSO_4$$

Properties:

1. Molar Mass of hydrogen peroxide is 34.0147gm/mol.

2. Appearance of hydrogen peroxide is very light blue in colour and colourless in solution.

3. Density of hydrogen peroxide is $1.463 gm/cm^3$.

4. Melting Point of hydrogen peroxide is $0.43°C$, 273 K, $31°F$.

5. Boiling Point of hydrogen peroxide is $150.2°C$, 423 K, $302°F$.

6. Hydrogen peroxide is Soluble in ether; miscible with water.

7. Acidity (pKa)of hydrogen peroxide is 11.62.

chemical reaction:

1. **As Reducing Agent:** When hydrogen peroxide reacts with silver oxide, it gives a black precipitate of reduced silver.

$$Ag_2O\downarrow + H_2O_2 \rightarrow 2Ag\downarrow + H_2O + O_2$$

2. **Action of Heat:** When dilute solutions of hydrogen peroxide are heated $100°C$, it rapidly undergoes decomposition to release oxygen.

$$2H_2O_2 \leftrightarrow 2H_2O + O_2$$

3. **As Oxidising Agent:** When ferrous sulphate undergoes oxidation with dilute sulphuric acid, the ferrous solution turns yellow from green.

$$2Fe^{++} + 2H^+ + H_2O_2 \rightarrow 2Fe^{+3} + H_2O$$

4. **Action with Black Lead Sulphide:** When black-coloured lead sulphide reacts with hydrogen peroxide, it gives white-coloured lead sulphate.

$$PbS\downarrow + 4H_2O_2 \rightarrow PbSO_4 + 4H_2O$$

Medicinal Uses:

1. It is used as a disinfectant, anti-infective, and deodorant. The oxygen released has antimicrobial action that is reduced in the presence of organic matter.

2. It is used as a mild oxidizing antiseptic at concentrations up to 6% to clean wounds and ulcers. It destroys most of the pathogenic bacteria, **e.g.,** Escherichia coli, Staphylococcus aureus, and typhoid bacilli.

3. Around 1.5% of its solution is used as a deodorant gargle and as a mouthwash for treating acute stomatitis.

4. It is used to clean septic sockets and root canals in dentistry.

5. It is available as ear-drops used for removing wax. The effervescent action of H2O2 removes dirt, bacteria, and debris from the wound surface or areas which are difficult to reach, **e.g.,** the ear canal.

Q.19. Write the preparation, properties and uses of Chlorinated lime.

Chlorinated Lime [$CaOCl(Cl)H_2O$]: Chlorinated lime (molecular weight 142.98) is also known as calc hypochlorite and bleaching powder. A sample of it should not have than 30.0% w/w of available chlorine.

Method of Preparation:

The reaction of chlorine with calcium hydroxide gives chlorinated lime. The slaked lime is spread on shelves in an appropriate container Subsequently, the chlorine gas is introduced from the top of the chamber and is permitted to pass through the contents of the shelves. This operation is carried out at 25°C and thus the formation of calcium chloride is reduced When the absorption of chlorine is completed, powdered lime is driven in the chamber in order to absorb the extra chlorine.

$$Ca(OH)_2 + Cl_2 \rightarrow Ca(OCl).Cl + H_2O$$

The process involved in the preparation is slightly complex. The basic chlorides (**e.g.,** CaCl2 Ca(OH), H_2O) and basic hypochlorite (**e.g.,** Ca(OCI), 2Ca(OH)2) are the primary product in this preparation. The basic hypochlorite (calcium hypochlorite) further reacts with chlorine and is changed. The commercial samples contain small fractions of calcium chlorate.

Assay:

In the presence of acid, the chlorinated lime usually liberates the available chlorine. The chlorine liberated when a substance reacts with acids is the available chlorine. Iodine is produced when the liberated chlorine reacts with potassium iodide. The quantity of iodine produced is estimated by titrating it with **0.1N $Na_2S_2O_3$**.

$$Ca(OCl)\ Cl + 2CH_3COOH \rightarrow Ca(CH_3COO)_2 + H_2O + Cl_2$$
$$Cl_2 + 2KI \rightarrow 2KCl + I_2$$
$$2Na_2S_2O_3 + I_2 \rightarrow 2NaI + Na_2S_4O_6$$

The steps involved in the assay of chlorinated lime are:

1. 4gm of accurately weighed bleaching powder is triturated with consecutive smaller quantities of water.

2. The resultant solution is to a titration flask and the volume is made up to the mark.

3. 100ml of the resultant suspension is in to a flask and treated with 3gm of KI solution.

4. This solution is acidified by adding 5ml of acetic acid and iodine is liberated.

5. The liberated iodine is titrated with 0.1N sodium thiosulphate, using starch mucilage as an indicator.

Each ml of 0.1N thiosulphate 0.003545gm of available chlorine

Properties:

1. It is a dull white powder with a characteristic odour.

2. After being exposed to air it absorbs moisture and decomposes slowly.

3. It is partially soluble in both water and alcohol.

4. After the bleaching powder is dissolved in water the hypochlorite moves into the solution and shows bleaching as well as oxidizing properties. A few important reactions of beaching powder are:

$$2NH_3 + 3ClO^- \rightarrow N_2\uparrow + 3Cl^- + 3H_2O$$
$$H2O2 + ClO^- \rightarrow O_2\uparrow + Cl^- + H_2O$$
$$HClO + HCl \rightarrow Cl_2\uparrow + H_2O$$
$$HClO + H^+ + 2I^- \rightarrow Cl^-\uparrow + I_2 + H_2O$$

Medicinal Uses:

1. Chlorinated lime is used as bleaching agent.

2. It is used as an antiseptic.

3. It is used as a cleaning solution for patients.

4. It is used as a disinfectant.

5. It is used locally in scarlet fever, diphtheria, aphthae, and gangrene.

6. It is used as internally in scrofula, typhus, malignant scarlet fever, syphilis, etc.

Q.20. Write the preparation, properties and uses of Iodine and its preparations.

Iodine (I_2) and its Preparations: Iodine (molecular weight 126.90), with symbol **'I'** and atomic number 53, is a naturally-occurring element in combined state. It is a single isotope with 74 neutrons. Among all the halogens, Iodine is the second least reactive and the second most electropositive halogen.

Methods of Preparation:

1. **From Seaweed:** The organic matter is removed from seaweed by drying and burning it. The ash obtained is extracted with water. Now the solution is concentrated and cooled which results in the deposition of the less soluble salts of alkaline metals, leaving behind the iodides in the solution. After the crystals are removed, the concentrated liquor is heated with manganese dioxide and concentrated sulphuric acid. Iodine is distilled off, condensed, and purified by sublimation.

$$2I^- + MnO_2 + 4H^+ \rightarrow 2H_2O + Mn^{++} + I_2$$

2. **From Chile Saltpetre:** Iodine occurs as sodium iodate $(NaIO_3)$ in Chile saltpetre and after the crystallisation of saltpetre it is left in the solution. The solution is treated with calculated quantity of sodium bisulphite wooden vats to bring about the following reactions:

a. **When bisulphite acts as an acid salt:**

$$NaIO_3 + NaHSO_3 \rightarrow Na_2SO_3 + HIO_3$$

b. **When it acts as a reducing agent:**

$$HIO_3 + 3NaHSO_3 \rightarrow 3NaHSO_4 + HI$$

c. **When hydroiodic acid reduces iodic acid:**

$$HIO_3 + 5HI \rightarrow 3H_2O + 3I_2$$

The obtained Iodine is filtered, washed, dried, and purified sublimation.

3. **From Oil-Field Waters:** Extracting iodine from oilfield water can be done as illustrated in the equation. Iodides in the water are oxidised thus, converting the inorganic iodine into its molecular form.

$$2NaI + 2NaNO_2 + 2H_2SO_4 \rightarrow I_2 + 2Na_2SO_4 + 2NO_2\uparrow + 2H_2O$$

Properties:

1. Iodine occurs as heavy, greyish black granules or plates, having metallic lustre and a characteristic odour.

2. It is freely soluble in carbon disulphide, chloroform, ether, and carbon tetrachloride

3. It is sparingly soluble in water and glycerine; soluble in alcohol and solution of iodides.

Chemical reaction:

1. It gives a black explosive powder of nitrogen trioxide by reacting with liquor ammonia.

$$2NH_3 + 3I_2 \rightarrow NI_3 + 3HI$$

2. It forms alkyl iodides by reacting with organic compounds.

$$CH_4 + I_2 \rightarrow CH_3I + HI$$

3. It forms potassium periodide by getting dissolved in potassium iodide solution.

$$KI + I \rightarrow KI_3$$

4. It turns starch solution blue by reacting with it.

5. It gets oxidised to iodate by reacting with strong oxidising agents.

$$3I_2 + 5KClO_3 + 3H_2O \rightarrow 5KCl + 6HIO_3$$

Medicinal Uses:

1. It is one of the best antiseptics.
2. It is a non-selective bactericide and sporicidal active against bacteria, fungi, yeast, protozoa, and viruses.
3. Its 2% solution in glycerol is used as a throat paint.
4. Iodine forms a complex with the amino groups present in the tissue, so as to form iodophors. Iodine is slowly liberated from iodophors to maintain a sustained action.

Iodine Preparation:

1. Aqueous Iodine Solution
2. Povidone Iodine

3. Sodium Iodide (NaI)

1. Aqueous Iodine Solution: Aqueous iodine solution contains about 5.0% w/v of Iodine (4.9-5.1%) and 10% w/v of potassium iodide (9.8-10.2%) in purified water.

Method of Preparation: Firstly, potassium iodide and iodine are dissolved in 100ml water with constant shaking or trituration. By adding adequate quantity of purified water volume is made up to 1000ml.

Properties: Aqueous iodine solution occurs as a transparent, brown liquid with a characteristic smell of iodine.

Chemical reactions:

1. It oxidises iron to form ferrous iodide.
$$Fe + I_3 \rightarrow FeI_3$$

2. Strong oxidising agents oxidise iodine to iodate, as illustrated with potassium chlorate.
$$3I_2 + 5KClO_3 + 3H_2O \rightarrow 5KCl + 6HIO_3$$

3. In base, iodine forms both iodide and iodate salts with ammonium hydroxide solution.
$$3I_2 + 6NH_4OH + 5NH_4I \rightarrow NH_4IO_3 + 3H_2O$$

Medicinal Uses:

Aqueous iodine solution can be administered internally as a good source of iodine. It shows germicidal as well as fungicidal It does not cause any irritation on cuts or wounds if given as a tincture.

2. Povidone Iodine: Iodine forms a complex with povidone to form povidone iodine. Povidone iodine (molecular weight 40,000) is a polymer and is also known as polyvinylpyrrolidone (PVP). After the povidone iodine complex is dried at 105°C to a constant weight, it should have at least 9.0% and minimum 120% of available I_2 (iodine).

Povidone-iodine is an example of class of iodophor compounds. Iodophor are iodine complexes with carrier organic molecules, and function a solubilising agent. These complexes gradually release iodine into p solution. Iodophors were developed in order to prepare less irritating iodine products with equivalent antibacterial property.

Method of Preparation:

Povidone-iodine is prepared by heating povidone with elemental iodine in the presence of a small quantity of water. It has at least 9.0% and minimum 12% of available iodine.

Properties:

1. It is a yellowish-brown amorphous powder with a slight characteristic odour.
2. It is soluble in both water and alcohol, but is insoluble in organic solvents.
3. Its aqueous solution is acidic in nature.
4. The structure of iodine complex with polyvinylpyrrolidone is not clearly known. However, by studying the UV absorption spectrum of iodine, it appears like a chemical linkage rather than a simple physical entrapment.

Medicinal Uses:

Povidone iodine is active against a wide range of microorganisms like gram-positive and gram-negative bacteria, fungi, viruses, protozoa, and yeast. Its solutions are frequently used for surgical scrubs, de-germ the skin prior to injection. It is also used for disinfection of wounds, burns. abrasions, and lacerations.

3. Sodium Iodide (NaI): Sodium iodide (molecular weight 1499) is a white crystalline salt. It is used in radiation detection, treatment of iodine deficiency and as a reactant in the Finkelstein reaction.

Method of Preparation:

Sodium iodide is prepared by the reaction of iodine with sodium hydroxide. Sodium iodate is formed when excess of iodine is added to the solution of sodium hydroxide, which is reduced by carbon to sodium iodide.

Properties:

1. It is a colourless, white, crystalline powder.
2. It remains stable in dry air but generally degrades and develops a brown colour on storage.
3. An aqueous solution of sodium iodide is either neutral or weakly alkaline to litmus

Medicinal Uses:

1. It is used in the treatment of thyroid disorder.
2. It is employed as a fibrinolytic agent in leprosy.

UNIT – 4
MISCELLANEOUS AGENTS

Q.1. Define following terms with suitable examples.

1. **Expectorants**
2. **Emetics**
3. **Haematinics**
4. **Antidotes**
5. **Astringents**

1. Expectorants: An **expectorant** is a therapeutic agent that helps to expel mucus, cell debris, and foreign particles out from the respiratory tract (lungs, bronchi, and trachea). **Example:** Potassium iodide, Guaifenesin is the most commonly used expectorant.

2.Emetics: An **emetic** (**e.g.,** syrup of ipecac) is a therapeutic preparation used to induce vomiting when any undesirable substance has been ingested. These agents help to expel toxic substances from the body immediately; therefore, many toxic and easily digestible poisonous products such as rat poison contain an emetic. **Example:** Copper sulphate, Apomorphine, etc.

3.Haematinics: Haematinics are the drugs used to enhance the concentration of haemoglobin (iron) in blood or used to cure blood disorders, like iron- deficiency anaemia. **Example:** Ferrous sulphate, Ferrous gluconate.

4.Antidotes are therapeutic agents used to neutralise the effects of a poison. Such substances are used to remove poison from the stomach by emesis induction or gastric lavage, for example, activated charcoal is administered orally to reduce absorption of poison. **Example:** Sodium thiosulphate, Copper sulphate.

5.Astringents precipitate proteins on the surface layer of skin and mucous membranes, resulting to their shrinkage. They are applied topically over damaged skin or mucous membrane of GIT, including mouth Precipitated protein along with the astringent forms a protective layer on skin surface. **Example:** Zinc sulphate, Potash alum.

Q.2. Write a note on Expectorant with characteristic and examples.

Expectorants: Expectorants or mucolytic agents are used to expel sputum from the respiratory tract either by enhancing the fluidity of sputum (i.e., reducing viscosity) or by increasing the volume of fluids to be expelled by coughing through the respiratory tract.

These agents are used to clear thick mucus from the respiratory pathway, including the lungs, bronchi, and trachea; thus, providing relief from respiratory tract disorders. They perform their action by hydrolysing the glycosaminoglycans, thus, reducing the viscosity of mucin possessing secretions. The concentration of mucoproteins influences the viscosity of mucous secretions in the lungs. Guaifenesin is the most common example of expectorant that acts by reducing the mucous viscosity, thus, facilitating the drainage of mucous from lungs as well as lubricating the irritated respiratory tract.

Characteristics:

1. It should be non-toxic,
2. It should not cause any allergy
3. It should also act as a mucolytic agent
4. It should increase the secretions from bronchi and also reduce its viscosity.

Classification:(Based on the mechanism of action)

1. Saline expectorants
2. Stimulant expectorants
3. Mucolytic expectorants
4. Anodyne / sedative expectorants

1. Saline Expectorants: These help in promoting the amount of bronchial secretion by salt-action.

2. Stimulant Expectorants: These help in stimulating bronchial glands and increase secretions from them. These also help in repairing and healing bronchial mucosa.

3. Mucolytic Expectorants: These help in reducing viscosity, and facilitate thinning and loosening of bronchial secretions. These act effectively when the mucus is purulent, i.e., infected.

4. Anodyne/Sedative Expectorants: These help in increasing the secretions and productivity of sputum. These also help in protecting mucosa and reduce recurrent coughing.

Examples:

1. Potassium iodide,
2. Ammonium chloride,
3. Ammonium acetate,
4. Ammonium carbonate,
5. Ammonium acetate, etc.

Q.3. Give Preparation, Properties, Uses and Assay of Ammonium chloride.

Ammonium Chloride (NH_4Cl): Ammonium chloride (molecular weight 53.50) is having not less than 99.5% of ammonium chloride which has been calculated with respect to the reference substance dried for 4 hours over silica gel.

Methods of Preparation:

1. On a commercial scale, it can be obtained by reacting ammonia gas with hydrochloric acid, and evaporating the resultant solution to dryness.

$$NH_3 + HCl \rightarrow NH_4Cl$$

The purification of the residue obtained is done by sublimation or crystallisation. Sublimation of volatile iron salt is prevented by mixing salt of 5% calcium phosphate at the time of purification. Generally, the sublimation is performed in cast iron pots which are lined with fire clay having a dome of glass.

2. It can also be prepared by reacting ammonia gas liquors with lime by the liberation of ammonia which is passed through hydrochloric acid.

Assay:

Earlier precipitation titration using Volhard's method was preferred for assaying ammonium chloride.

The steps involved in this assay were:

1. Accurately weighed 0.2gm of NH_4Cl was dissolved in 40ml of water.
2. The solution obtained was acidified with 3ml of nitric acid.
3. Further, 50ml of N/10 silver nitrate and 5ml of nitrobenzene were added to this acidic solution and shaken vigorously.
4. The excess of silver nitrate was titrated with N/10 ammonium thiocyanate, using 2ml of ferric ammonium sulphate as an indicator.

$$NH_4Cl + AgNO_3 \rightarrow NH_4NO_3 + AgCl$$
Each ml of 0.1N $AgNO_3$ = 0.005349gm of NH_4Cl

Currently, acid-base titration is preferred for assay of ammonium chloride. This method is comparatively simple and economic as it does not require silver nitrate.

The steps involved are:

1. Accurately weighed 0.1gm of NH_4Cl is taken in a conical flask.

2. 50ml of water is added to the flask to dissolve the sample.

3. 5ml of neutralised formaldehyde solution is again added to the above solution.

4. There be a possibility that the formaldehyde solution undergoes atmospheric oxidation and forms a small amount of formic acid. This acid should be neutralised by titrating with dilute sodium hydroxide solution, using phenolphthalein as an indicator.

5. Any additional amount of alkali should not be present in this reagent.

6. The resultant solution is left undisturbed for a few minutes.

7. The hydrochloric acid liberated is titrated with standard sodium hydroxide solution, using phenolphthalein as an indicator.

Each ml of 0.IN sodium hydroxide consumed = 0.005349gm of NH_4Cl

The principle involved is that ammonium chloride hydrolyses into ammonium hydroxide (base) and hydrogen chloride (acid). This hydrolysis is catalysed by formaldehyde which does so by fixing ammonia and forming hexamine. Finally, the acid is titrated using an alkali.

The reactions are summarised below:

$$NH_4Cl + H_2O \rightarrow NH_4OH + HCl$$
$$NH_4OH + 6CH_2O \rightarrow C_6H_{12}N_4 + 10H_2O$$
$$HCl + NaOH \rightarrow NaCl + H_2O$$

Ammonium chloride assay relies on the principle of titration. The ammonium chloride solution attains acidic properties on adding formaldehyde solution into it. Thus, the solution can be titrated using phenolphthalein indicator.

Properties:

1. It is a colourless or white, crystalline or course powder.
2. It is odourless with a cooling saline taste.
3. It is freely soluble in water and glycerine, but sparingly soluble in alcohol.
4. It is slightly hygroscopic.
5. Freshly prepared aqueous solution of ammonium chloride is neutral, but it rapidly becomes acidic on storing due to hydrolysis.
6. It is incompatible with the carbonates of alkaline earth metals, lead salts, and with alkalis.

Medicinal Uses:

1. It regulates acid-base equilibrium between the body fluids. Ammonia formed by deamination of amino acids is exerted in the kidney and in this process sodium ions are retained.
2. Ammonium cations are converted into urea to exert a diuretic effect during this process proton H and CT ions are also formed. Carbon dioxide gas and water is formed by the reaction of hydrogen ion with bicarbonate.

During the process, bicarbonate ions are lost and alkali reserve of the body is reduced. On continuous use increase in urine acidity and metabolic acidosis is produced.

3. Small doses of ammonium chloride act as a mild expectorant and diaphoretic. This is because local irritation stimulates secretion of respiratory tract and also makes the mucus less viscous. Hence, the salts of ammonium chloride and ammonium carbonate are used in expectorant

Q.4. Give Preparation, Properties, and Uses of Potassium iodide.

Potassium Iodide (KI): Potassium iodide (molecular weight 166) is not having less than 99% KI which has been calculated with respect to the dried reference substance at 105°C up to a constant weight.

Methods of Preparation:

1. It can be prepared by treating iodine with moist iron filling to form ferro-ferric iodide ($FeI_2.FeI_2$) which undergoes decomposition with potassium carbonate.

$$FeI_2 + I_2 \rightarrow FeI_2.FeI_3$$
$$FeI_2.FeI_3 + 4K_2CO_3 \rightarrow 8KI + FeO.Fe_2O_3 + 4CO_2 \uparrow$$

The resultant product, i.e., a ferrosoferric oxide is filtered and the filtrate is concentrated to yield potassium iodide salt. It can be purified by the process of recrystallisation.

$$6KOH + 3I_2 \rightarrow 5KI + KIO_3 + 2H_2O$$
$$KIO_3 + 3C \rightarrow KI + 3CO \uparrow$$

2. It can also be prepared by the reaction of excess of iodine with potassium hydroxide solution to form potassium iodate and

iodide. Reduction of potassium iodate to potassium iodide occurs in the presence of carbon.

Properties:

1. It is an odourless, transparent or opaque salt with saline bitter taste.
2. In moist air, KI is deliquescent. It is soluble in alcohol, water and glycerine.
3. When added to water the temperature of the resultant solution gets lowered.
4. This aqueous solution of potassium iodide forms KI3, KL, etc., along with iodine.

Medicinal Uses:

1. It is used as an expectorant due to the presence of iodide ions. Its expectorant action is rapid for producing bronchial fluid for diluting the sputum.
2. It is supplied either in solution or in tablet form. Recommended dose is about 0.3gm. The KI tablets are enteric coated for masking the bitter metallic taste.
3. It is used as a source of potassium and iodine.
4. It also acts as a stabiliser in the formulations of iodine solutions. It also acts as a reagent in pharmacy.

Q.5. What are emetics? Mention their characteristics and examples.

Emetics: A drug which aids in emptying emetic. Some of these drugs are inorganic compounds (**e.g.,** antimony potassium tartrate) and aid in removing fluid from the respiratory tract by directly stimulating secretion of respiratory tract. This is because emetics are chief component of most of the cough syrups.

The different mechanisms by which emetics act upon are:

1. Emetics like morphine, ergot, and digitalis glycosides stimulate the chemoreceptor trigger zone present in the postrema of the medulla oblangata.
2. Emetics like zinc sulphate, copper sulphate, and sodium chloride act by irritating the GIT.
3. Emetics like veratrum stimulate the ganglion of the vagus.
4. Some of the emetics stimulate receptors in the heart and in the CNS to the brain stem.

The use of emetics is avoided in patients who are unconscious, in coma, in a state of depression or shock, with severe heart disease, tuberculosis, etc.

Characteristics:

1. Non-toxic,
2. Non-interactive with other drugs,
3. Devoid of side effects,
4. Non-irritant, and
5. Short onset of action.

Examples:

1. Copper sulphate,
2. Sodium potassium tartarate,
3. Antimony potassium tartarate,
4. Ipecacuanha,
5. Apomorphine, etc.

Q.6. Give Preparation, Properties, Uses and Assay of Copper sulphate.

Copper Sulphate ($CuSO_4.5H_2O$): Copper sulphate (molecular weight 249.7) should contain 98.5-101% of$CuSO_4.5H_2O$

Methods of Preparation:

1. It is prepared by either roasting sulphide ore (containing copper) in the presence of air or heating copper and sulphur in a furnace. A mixture of copper sulphate and copper oxide is obtained which is further treated with dilute sulphuric acid. The resulting solution is filtered, concentrated, and allowed to undergo crystallisation.

2. It can also be prepared by the reaction of granulated copper and sulphuric acid in the presence of air.

$$2Cu + 2H_2OSO_4 + O_2 \rightarrow CuSO_4 + 2H_2O$$

Assay: The underlying principle of assaying copper sulphate is that $CuSO_4$ and KI react together to form an unstable cupric iodide. Further the cupric oxide decomposes to yield Cu_2I_2 and freed iodine.

The steps involved in the assay of copper sulphate are:

1. A suitable amount of copper sulphate is weighed and dissolved in water.
2. KI and acetic acid are added in the above solution.
3. Iodine is obtained which is titrated with standard sodium thiosulphate solution, using starch as an indicator.
4. The titration is continued till the faint blue colour of solution appears.
5. 2gm of KCNS (potassium thiocyanate) is added to the solution and titration is performed till the blue colour vanishes.

   1ml of 0.1N Na2S303= 0.02497gm of $CuSO_4.5H_2O$

Properties:

1. Copper sulphate exists as deep blue coloured, triclinic crystals of pentahydrate or blue crystalline granules or powder.
2. When exposed to dry air it loses moisture, and thus a layer of white anhydrous salt forms on the crystals.
3. Copper sulphate is water soluble, and insoluble in alcohol.
4. Its aqueous solutions are acidic to litmus paper.

Medicinal Uses:

1. Earlier it was utilised as emetics (300mg in 30ml water) which rapidly activates the vomiting centre, thus, used in chemical poisoning.
2. At the present time it is used as an astringent and a fungicide (in 1-5% concentration) meant for external application.

3. It is also a constituent of Benedict and Fehling reagents.

Q.7. Give Preparation, Properties, Uses of Sodium potassium tartrate.

SODIUM POTASSIUM TARTRATE ($KNaC_4H_4O_6.4H_2O$): The molecular weight of sodium potassium tartrate is 282.2. It should not have less than 99% and not more 104% of $KNaC_4H_4O_6.4H_2O$

Method of Preparation:

It can be prepared by neutralising of sodium carbonate with potassium bitartrate. Then the solution is boiled for a while and heated at temperature of 60°C for the completion of reaction and for the neutrality adjustment. The solution is concentrated to crystallisation and then filtered.

$$2KHC_4H_4O_6 + Na_2CO_3.H_2O + 6H_2O \rightarrow 2KNaC_4H_4O_6.4H_2O + 6CO_2 \uparrow$$

Properties:

1. In slightly warm and dry air, it loses its water content rapidly.
2. Generally, the crystals are coated with a white powder.
3. It is tartar with minimum concentration of tartaric acid and has about 68% of total content. Firstly, it is dissolved in water or mother liquor with the previous batch preparation. With hot caustic soda it can be saponified at pH 8. Activated charcoal has discolouring properties, and can be purified before filtering the solution. The resultant filtrate is evaporated at 100°C, and is passed through the granulators on which the

Seignette's salt is used to crystallise on slow cooling. By centrifugation method, the salt can be easily separated out along with the washing of the granules. It can be dried in a rotatory furnace, and before its packaging it can be sieved.

Medicinal Uses:

1. It is used as an emetic for removing the toxic substances from the body in case of poisoning.
2. It is used as a saline cathartic.

Q.8. Define Haematinics with examples. Give Preparation, Properties, Uses and Assay of Ferrous sulphate.

Haematinics: Haematinics are the drugs used to increase the concentration of haemoglobin(iron) in blood or used to cure anaemia mainly due to iron deficiency. These agents are required for the formation of blood.

Examples:

1. Ferrous sulphate,
2. Ferrous gluconate,
3. Ferric ammonium citrate, etc.

FERROUS SULPHATE ($FeSO_4.7H2O$)

Ferrous sulphate (molecular weight 278) used as a haematic should have 20% Fe. It is also known as green vitriol.

Methods of Preparation:

1. It can be prepared by dissolving iron in excess of dilute sulphuric acid which produces effervescence. Thereafter, the solution is filtered, concentrated and cooled. Filtration is carried out at room temperature to separate the green coloured crystals. In the above processes, ferrous sulphate should not be exposed to air as it undergoes rapid oxidation when comes in contact with moist air. As a result, ferric sulphate forms a brownish yellow coating over the crystals.

$$Fe + H_2SO_4 \rightarrow FeSO_4 + H_2 \uparrow$$

The mercurous chloride is reduced to mercuric chloride by ferrous sulphate in the presence of light.

$$2HgCl_2 + 2Fe_2+ \rightarrow Hg_2Cl_2 + 2Fe^{3+} + 2Cl^-$$

Evolution of carbon dioxide occurs when a reaction takes place between ferrous sulphate and sodium carbonate solution.

$$FeSO_4 + Na_2CO_3 \rightarrow FeCO_3 + Na_2SO_4$$
$$FeCO_3 + H_2O \rightarrow Fe(OH)_2 + CO_2$$

For Fe^{2+} and SO_4^{2-}, ferrous sulphate shows different characteristic tests.

2. It can also be prepared when iron pyrites are exposed to air and moisture, giving the following reaction:

$$2FeS_2 + 7O_2 + 2H_2O \rightarrow 2FeSO_4 + 2H_2SO_4$$

Assay: Ferrous sulphate is assayed by redox reaction in which N/10 potassium permanganate solution is reacted with dilute H_2SO_4.

The steps involved in the assay are:

1. 1gm of ferrous sulphate is weighed and dissolved in 20ml of dilute H_2SO_4

2. The resultant solution is titrated with 0.IN KMnO4, as shown below:

   $2FeSO_4+2KMnO_4 + 4H_2SO_4 \rightarrow K_2SO_4 + 2MnSO_4 + Fe_2(SO_4)_3 + 4H_2O$

   Each ml of N/10 KMnO4 ≡ 0.0291g of $FeSO_4.7H_2O$

Another assay method of ferrous sulphate involves the following steps:

1. 1gm of ferrous sulphate is weighed and taken in a conical flask.

2. 30ml of water and 20ml of dilute sulphuric acid are added in the flask to dissolve ferrous sulphate.

3. The resultant solution is titrated with standard 0.1M ceric ammonium nitrate solution, using ferroin sulphate solution as an indicator.

4. The titration is continued till the red colour changes to light blue.

   Each ml of 0.1M ceric ammonium sulphate ≡ 0.0278g of ferrous sulphate heptahydrate.

Properties:

1. **Appearance:** Pale, bluish green crystals or granules,
2. **Odour:** Odourless,
3. **Taste:** Saline and styptic (astringent or bitter),
4. **Solubility:** Soluble in water (43.5gm in 100gm of water at 150°C),

5. **Acidic Nature:** Its solution is acidic to litmus at pH about 3.7.

6. **Crystal Properties:** Crystals undergo oxidation when comes in contact with air, forming brown patches of sulphate due to efflorescent nature,

Chemical properties:

1. It undergoes complete dehydration when heated at 300°C and in the absence of air it shows white colour. On further heating, the anhydrous solid produces sulphur dioxide, sulphur trioxide, and ferric oxide salts by undergoing decomposition.

$$FeSO_4.7H_2O \rightarrow FeSO_4 + 7H_2O$$

$$2FeSO_4 \rightarrow Fe_2O_3 + SO_2 + SO_3$$

2. It undergoes rapid oxidation and forms ferric effective reducing agent. It also reduces potassium permanganate sulphate; thus, it is potassium dichromate, etc.

$$6FeSO_4 + K_2Cr_2O_7 + 7H_2SO_4 \rightarrow K_2SO_4 + Cr_2(SO4)_3 + 3Fe_2(SO_4)_3 + 7H_2O$$

$$10FeSO_4 + 2KMnO_4 + 8H_2SO_4 \rightarrow K_2SO_4 + 2MnSO_4 + 5Fe_2(SO_4)_3 + 8H_2O$$

3. Evolution of carbon dioxide occurs by reacting sodium carbonate solution with ferrous sulphate.

$$FeSO_4 + Na_2CO_3 \rightarrow FeCO_3 + Na_2SO_4$$
$$FeCO_3 + 2H_2O \rightarrow Fe(OH)_2 + CO_2$$

4. Black coloured nitroso-ferrous sulphate $(FeSO_4.NO)$ is formed by the reaction between ferrous dichromate into green.

$$2FeSO_4 + H_2SO_4 + NO_2 \rightarrow Fe_2(SO_4)_3 + H_2O + NO$$

5. Being a reducing agent, it decolourises potassium permanganate and converts potassium dichromate into green.

6. It combines with alkali metal sulphates and forms double salts (R_2SO_4. $FeSO_46H_2O$).

It forms ferrous ammonium sulphate [$FeSO_4.(NH_4)_2SO_4.6H_2O$], i.e., Mohr's salt, with ammonium sulphate.

Medicinal uses:

1. It is a haematinic preparation most widely used for treating iron-deficiency anaemia.
2. It enhances formation of haemoglobin.

Q.9. Give Preparation, Properties, and Uses of Ferrous gluconate.

Haematinics: Haematinics are the drugs used to increase the concentration of haemoglobin(iron) in blood or used to cure anaemia mainly due to iron deficiency. These agents are required for the formation of blood.

Examples:

1. Ferrous sulphate,
2. Ferrous gluconate,

FERROUS GLUCONATE ($C_{12}H_{22}FeO_{14}.2H_2O$) (12% Fe)

The molecular weight of ferrous gluconate is 482.18. A given sample of it should not have less than 95% of $C_{12}H_{22}O_{14}Fe$ Methods of Preparation

Methods of Preparation:

1. By the metathesis reaction between hot solutions of calcium gluconate and ferrous sulphate, insoluble calcium sulphate and ferrous gluconate are obtained. The resultant hot mixture is filtered to expel calcium sulphate and the filtrate is evaporated to give crystal-like structures.

$$FeSO_4 + [COO^--(CHOH)_4-CH2OH]_2 + Ca^{2+} \rightarrow [COO^--(CHOH)_4-CH2OH]_2 + Ca^{2+} + CaSO_4$$

2. Freshly prepared ferrous carbonate is heated with suitable concentration of gluconic acid in aqueous solution to produce ferrous gluconate.

$$FeCO_3 + H_2O + [COO^--(CHOH)_4-CH2OH]_2 \rightarrow [COO^--(CHOH)_4-CH2OH]_2 + Fe^{2+} + 2H_2O + CO_2$$

Properties:

1. **Appearance:** Yellowish grey powder.
2. **Odour:** Odour of burnt sugar.
3. **Solubility:** Soluble in cold water (1gm in 5ml water) and insoluble in alcohol.
4. **pH:** Aqueous solution is acidic towards litmus. The sequence of colours depends upon the pH value (pH 2 light yellow; pH 4.5 brown; pH 7 green).
5. **Stability:** When comes in contact with air, it starts oxidising slowly to ferric form. It is also affected in the presence of light.

Medicinal uses:

1. It is formulated in tablet dosage form and is administered orally in case of iron deficiency.

2. It is also used in elixir form.

Q.10. Explain Poison and Antidote. Classify them with suitable examples. Give Preparation, Properties, Uses and Assay of Sodium thiosulphate.

Poison and Antidote: Agents used to neutralise the effect of a poison are known as antidotes. In case of acute poisoning, mostly the patients need symptomatic and supportive therapy. When activated charcoal is administered orally, it helps in the reduction of poison absorption. Such substances are used to remove poison from the stomach by emesis induction or gastric lavage.

The techniques (such as forced diuresis, haemodialysis, or hemoperfusion) used to remove poisons from the body are effective only for limited number of poisons.

Therefore, antidotes are used in specific conditions which are very effective for saving the life of people. Uses of such drugs are important for symptomatic and supportive treatment of poisoning.

Classification: (On the basis of Mode of action)
1. Chemical antidotes
2. Physiological antidotes
3. Mechanical antidotes

1. Chemical Antidotes: These antidotes are used to alter the chemical nature of the poison, **e.g.,** sodium thiosulphate converts toxic cyanide to non-toxic thiocyanate, and sodium calcium edetate forms chelates with toxic heavy metals.

2. Physiological Antidotes: These antidotes produce the reverse effect of poison, **e.g.,** conversion of haemoglobin into methaemoglobin by sodium nitrile to bind cyanide.

3. Mechanical Antidotes: These antidotes prevent the poison from getting absorbed into the body, **e.g.,** activated charcoal absorbs the poison before absorption by intestinal wall; and copper sulphate, magnesium sulphate and sodium mono hydrogen phosphate inactivates the toxic material and precipitate it by chelation as insoluble salts.

Examples:

1. Sodium thiosulphate,
2. Activated charcoal,
3. Sodium nitrite,
4. Sodium nitrile,
5. Copper sulphate, etc.

SODIUM THIOSULPHATE ($Na_2S_2O_3.5H_2O$): Sodium thiosulphate (molecular weight 248.18) contains not less than 99% and not more than 100.5% of $Na_2S_2O_3$.

Methods of Preparation:

1. Sodium sulphite solution, along with powdered sulphur is boiled gently in a porcelain dish for 20-30 minutes. As a result,

the sulphite gets oxidised to sodium thiosulphate. After evaporation to small bulk and on cooling, the solution deposits colourless crystal of the hydrate ($Na_2S_2O_3.5H_2O$), which is filtered, washed with slightly cold distilled water and dried.

$$Na_2S_2O_2 + S \rightarrow Na_2S_2O_3$$

2. In industries, it is produced from lighting gas formed in the coking of coal. Lighting gas contains hydrogen sulphide which is trapped by calcium hydroxide forming calcium sulphide.

$$Ca(OH)_2 + H_2S \rightarrow CaS + 2H_2O$$

Calcium sulphide undergoes hydrolysis to form calcium hydrosulphide.

$$CaS + 2H_2O \rightarrow Ca(OH)_2 + H_2S$$
$$2Ca(OH)_2 + 3H_2S \rightarrow CaS + Ca(SH)_2 + 4H_2O$$

Calcium hydrosulphide undergoes oxidation by the oxygen of air to form calcium thiosulphate;

$$Ca(SH)_2 + 2O_2 \rightarrow CaS_2O_3 + H_2O$$

Fusion of calcium thiosulphate with sodium sulphate or carbonate produces sodium thiosulphate;

$$CaS_2O_3 + Na_2CO_3 \rightarrow Na_2S_2O_3 + CaCO_3 \text{ (White)}$$

Evaporation of the solution produces sodium thiosulphate crystals.

3. It can be prepared by passing sulphur dioxide into sodium sulphide solution.

$$2Na_2S + 3SO_2 \rightarrow 2Na_2S_2O_3 + S$$

4. It can also be prepared by treating a mixture of sodium sulphide and sodium sulphite with iodine.

$$Na_2S + Na_2SO_3 + I_2 \rightarrow Na_2S_2O_3 + 2NaI$$

Assay: Sodium thiosulphate is assayed by dissolving 0.5gm of the dried sample in 30ml of water. The resultant solution is titrated with 0.IN iodine solution, using starch TS indicator.

Each ml of 0.1N iodine = 15.81mg of $Na_2S_2O_3$

Properties:

1. It is colourless, transparent crystals having a bitter salty taste.
2. It dissolves rapidly in water and is insoluble in alcohol.

Chemical reactions:

1. **Reducing Properties:** It possesses reducing properties due to the presence of S in a molecule. It reduces iodine to iodide (I^-), while sodium thiosulphate is oxidised by iodine to sodium tetrathionate.

$$2Na_2S2O_3 + I_2 \rightarrow 2NaI + Na_2S_4O_6$$

Chlorine is reduced to hydrogen chloride.

$$Cl_2 + Na_2S_2O_3 + H_2O \rightarrow 2HCl + S\downarrow + Na_2SO_4$$

With an excess of chlorine, the evolved sulphur oxidises to sulphuric acid.

$$S-3Cl_2+4H_2O \rightarrow H_2SO_4 + 6HCl$$

The overall reaction is;

$$4Cl_2 + Na_2S_2O_3 + 5H_2O \rightarrow 2NaHSO_4 + 8HCl$$

The use of sodium thiosulphate in the gas masks for chlorine based on this reaction. Absorption

2. **Stability:** It melts in its water of hydration at 56°C, loses its water of crystallisation at 215°C, and decomposes when

heated above 220°C. This decomposition gives sodium and sodium penta sulphide and finally sulphur, sulphur dioxide, and sodium sulphide.

$$4Na_2S_2O_3 \rightarrow 3Na_2SO_4 + Na_2S_5$$
$$Na_2S_5 \rightarrow Na_2S + 4S$$
$$Na_2S_5 + 4O_2 \rightarrow Na_2S + 4SO_4$$

With silver nitrate solution, a white precipitate of silver thiosulphate is formed which turns yellow. When allowed to stand, the precipitate becomes black under the influence of atmospheric moisture forming silver sulphide.

$$Na_2S_2O_3 + 2AgNO_3 \rightarrow Ag_2S_2O_3 + 2NaNO_3$$
$$Ag_2S_2O_3 \rightarrow Ag_2SO_3 + S$$
$$Ag_2SO_3 + S + H_2O \rightarrow Ag_2S + H_2SO_4$$

Sodium thiosulphate on reacting with iron (III) chloride solution forms purple coloured iron (III) thiosulphate. This colour rapidly disappears on reduction to a colourless iron (II) salt (FeS_2O_3 and FeS_4O_6).

$$2FeCl_3 + 3Na_2S_2O_3 \rightarrow 6NaCl + Fe_2(S_2O_3)_3$$
$$Fe_2(S_2O_3)_3 \rightarrow FeS_2O_3 + FeS_4O_6$$

3. It is used as an antidote in halogens, cyanogen, and hydrocyanic acid poisoning.

$$KCN + Na_2S_2O_3 \rightarrow KSCN + Na_2SO_3$$

The potassium thiocyanate obtained is less poisonous than potassium cyanide. Sodium thiosulphate can also be used in poisoning of arsenic, mercury and lead compounds as it converts them into sulphides which are non-poisonous.

Medicinal uses:

1. It is used in the treatment of cyanide poisoning with sodium nitrite,
2. It is used as an antioxidant, usually limited to iodides. Around 0.05% of sodium thiosulphate is used in KI solution. It is officially recognised as an antidote to cyanide poisoning.
3. It is also used as a topical antifungal agent.
4. Along with acids it is used for treating skin infections, like dermatophytosis and tinea *versicolour.*

Q.11. Give Preparation, Properties, and Uses of following.
a) Activated Charcoal
b) Sodium Nitrite

a) Activated Charcoal (Medicinal Charcoal): It is the residue obtained from the destructive distillation of various organic material treated to increase its adsorptive power.

Methods of Preparation:

1. **Activation of Charcoal:** The absorptive powers of charcoal increases by treating it with steam, air, carbon dioxide, oxygen, zinc chloride, sulphuric acid, or phosphoric acid, or a combination of some of these substances at temperature ranging from 500-900°C.

   In this process, the activating agent removes substances adsorbed on the charcoal and break down the granules of carbon into smaller ones having an increased surface area.

2. **Other Sources:** Sucrose, lactose, rice, starch, coconut pericarp, blood and various industrial wastes can be used for preparing charcoal.

3. **Destructive Distillation:** Commercially, it is obtained as a residue during destructive distillation of various organic matters or from burning of organic materials in a special manner. The so obtained coarse material is crushed and powdered.

Properties:

1. It is a fine, black, odourless, and tasteless powder, which is free from gritty matter.

2. It is insoluble in water and other organic solvents.

Chemical reactions:

1. **Decolourising Power:** Bromophenol blue (50ml of a 0.006% w solution) is taken in a 250ml flask and 0.1gm of charcoal sample is added and mixed in the flask.

   The solution is allowed to stand and filtered.

   The colour of the filtrate is not deeper than that of standard solution which is prepared by diluting 1ml of the solution of bromophenol blue to 50ml with alcohol (20%).

2. **Acid-Soluble Matter:**1gm of a sample of charcoal is heated on water-bath with 10ml of dilute H_2SO_4 and 20ml of water.

The sample is filtered and filtrate is evaporated to dryness. The weight of residue is not more than 25mg and sulphate ash not more than 5%.

Medicinal uses:

1. It dissolves rapidly in as an emergency antidote in many forms of poisoning.
2. It will adsorb alkaloids, NH_3, CO, CO_2, O_2, N_2, NO, and H_2.
3. Activated charcoal is used in filters of gas masks because of its ability to adsorb gases.
4. It is a preferred method for treatment of poisoning of virtually all drugs and chemicals except but amide. Acetaminophen, chlorpromazine, phenobarbital, strychnine, and sodium salicylate are some examples in which the charcoal is used as an antidote.

b) Sodium Nitrite ($NaNO_2$): Sodium nitrite has molecular weight of 68.99 and contains 97-101% of sodium nitrite which has been calculated with respect to the substance for 4 yours dried over silica gel.

Methods of preparation:

1. Other method involves reduction of sodium nitrate by lead (Pb), at a temperature of 450°C in iron pans.
2. One of the most effective method involves the absorption of NO (obtained during the catalytic oxidation of ammonia and

oxygen) by sodium carbonate solution. To crystallise the product the solution is concentrated.

$$2Na_2CO_3 + 4NO + O_2 \rightarrow 4NaNO_2 + 2CO_2$$

Properties:

1. It is colourless to slight yellowish crystals or white to slightly yellow granular powder.
2. It is odourless, saline in taste, and deliquescent.
3. It is soluble in water and sparingly insoluble in alcohol.
4. It deliquesces when exposed to air and gets oxidised to sodium nitrate.
5. Its aqueous solution shows alkaline properties.
6. It decomposes by acidification with dilute sulphuric acid.
7. It acts as a reducing agent and can get oxidised to nitrate in an acidic medium.
8. It also acts as an oxidising agent.

Medicinal uses:

1. It is used in cyanide poisoning methaemoglobin formation. It is given with sodium thiosulphate.
2. Nitrite ion also relaxes the smooth muscles of blood vessels showing its vasodilator action.
3. It is also used as preservative in food.

Q.12. Write a note on Astringents with classification and examples. Give Preparation, Properties, uses of Zinc Sulphate and Potash Alum.

Astringents: Substances which cause protein precipitation are known as astringents. They are applied topically on damaged skin, mouth and mucous membrane of gastrointestinal tract. Astringents and precipitated proteins form a protective layering.

This protective layer:

1. Protects against bacteria and infections,
2. Reduces exudation, and
3. Prevents capillary oozing when applied to bleeding areas.

Astringents shrink the mucous membranes or exposed tissues. They mildly coagulate the skin proteins, dry, harden, and protect the skin.

They also reduce the cell permeability because of their capability of precipitating proteins. The transcapillary movement of plasma proteins are restricted by astringents, thereby reducing local oedema, exudation, inflammation, and mucous secretion.

Classification:

1. **Vegetable Astringents:** These astringents are of two types:
   a. **Tannic acid:** It is a light-brown coloured powder, soluble in glycerine and alcohol.
   b. **Catechu:** It possesses astringent activity due to the presence of tannic acid.
2. **Metallic Astringents:** These astringents are of the following types:

a. **Aluminium salts:** Some important examples of this class of astringent are aluminium acetate, alum (aluminium potassium sulphate or aluminium ammonium sulphate), etc. It is used as a solution or powder. It damages enamel due to its acidic characters. Aluminium acetate has fewer irritant characters.

b. **Zinc salts:** Zinc chloride, zinc sulphate, and zinc oxide are used as astringents and antiseptics. They do not stain the teeth. Zinc sulphate possesses less irritant action to the oral mucosa as compared to zinc chloride. The activity of zinc oxide is weaker than other zinc salts.

c. **Ferric salts:** It is rarely used due to its ability of staining the teeth and damaging the enamel.

d. **Silver nitrate and Copper sulphate:** These astringents also stain the teeth.

Examples:

1. Zinc sulphate,
2. Potash alum,
3. Aluminium chloride,
4. Zinc chloride,
5. Zinc peroxide, etc.

Zinc Sulphate ($ZnSO_4.7H_2O$): Zinc sulphate (molecular weight 287.54), also known as white vitriol, either occurs naturally as mineral goslarite or can be synthesised by of zinc with sulphuric acid. It contains 55.6-61% of $ZnSO_4$ corresponding to 99.5-102% of the hydrated zinc sulphate ($ZnSO_4.7H_2O$).

Methods of Preparation:

1. It can be produced from its ore, i.e., zinc blend (ZnS) which is roasted. The sulphide gets converted into oxide which is treated with dilute sulphuric acid, resulting in the formation of zinc sulphate.

$$2ZnS + 3O_2 \rightarrow 2ZnO + 2SO_2$$
$$ZnO + H_2SO_4 \rightarrow ZnSO_4 + H_2O$$

2. It can also be prepared by directly reacting zinc with sulphuric acid.

$$Zn + 2H_2SO_4 \rightarrow ZnSO_4 + 2H_2O + SO2$$

Properties:

1. **Appearance:** Colourless, transparent crystals, prisms or needles, orgranular, crystalline powder.
2. **Odour:** Odourless.
3. **Taste:** Astringent and metallic taste.
4. **Solubility:** Highly soluble in 0.6 parts of water and 2.5 parts of glycerine, but insoluble in alcohol.
5. **Stability:** Effloresces in dry air.

Chemical reactions:

1. As zinc sulphate undergoes hydrolysis, a solution is obtained with pH around 5 and acidic to litmus paper.

$$ZnSO_4 + H2O \leftrightarrow Zn(OH)SO_4 + H^+$$

2. When Zn^{2+} reacts with sodium sulphide solution (an acidic medium), white precipitate of zinc sulphide is obtained from zinc salts (a distinction from other salts of heavy metals.)

$$ZnSO_4 + Na_2S \rightarrow ZnS \downarrow Na_2SO_4$$

3. When Zn^{2+} reacts with potassium ferrocyanide solution, a yellowish crystalline precipitate of a double salt is formed which is insoluble in acids but soluble in alkalis:

$$3ZnSO_4 + 2K_4[Fe(CN)_6] \rightarrow K_2Zn_3[Fe(CN)_6]_2 + 3K_2SO_4$$

4. When zinc oxide is roasted with cobalt nitrate, a characteristic colour is obtained.

$$ZnO + Co(NO_3)_2 \rightarrow CoZnO_2 + 2NO_2 \uparrow + 1/2\ O_2$$

Medicinal uses:

1. It is available in 0.1%, 0.25% and 0.5% solution to be used topically an antiseptic and ophthalmic astringent. It is often prescribed with boric acid in eye drops due to its acidic nature.

2. It is available in 0.1-0.5% solutions to be used in gynaecology for irrigation.

3. It can be orally administered for healing wounds.

4. It is used for treating acne, dandruff, ivy poisoning, lupus erythematosus, and a deodorant.

5. Orally it is used in the treatment of rheumatoid arthritis and acrodermatitis enter opathica.

6. It is a prompt emetic, i.e., it induces vomiting.

Potash Alum ($KAl(SO_4)_2.12H_2O$): Alum or potash alum is potassium aluminium sulphate with molecular weight 474.4. It is a double salt containing 99.5% or more of $KAl(SO_4)_2.12H_2O$

Method of Preparation:

Potash alum is prepared by mixing a concentrated solution of potassium sulphate with a hot solution of aluminium sulphate (present in an equivalent amount). After the resultant solution becomes concentrated and is cooled down, crystals of octahedral are separated out. Crystallisation preceded at a slower rate yields large crystals of octahedral.

$$K_2SO_4 + Al_2(SO_4) + 24H_2O \rightarrow 2KAl(SO_4)_2.12H_2O$$

Properties:

1. It exists as colourless, transparent, or granular crystals.
2. It exhibits a sweet astringent taste.
3. On heating slowly on water-bath temperature, it melts in its water of crystallisation.
4. It becomes anhydrous by losing its water of crystallisation at 200°C. It is water soluble and alcohol insoluble.

Medicinal uses:

1. It is used topically due to its astringent action.
2. It is used for preparing toxoids due to its ability to precipitate proteins.
3. It has antiseptic properties and is used as a local styptic.
4. It is utilised as a pharmaceutical aid.

UNIT – 5
<u>RADIOPHARMACEUTICALS</u>

Q.1. What is Radioactivity? Give the unit of Radioactivity.

Radioactivity: Radioactivity is defined as the nuclear instability which results in the radiation or emission of particles from the nuclei. There are various types of radiations, amongst them the most common types of radiations are alpha, beta, and gamma.

Radiopharmaceuticals are therapeutic molecules with radiolabelling. i.e., few atoms in these molecules are exchanged with their radioactive isotopes. Such radiolabelled molecules are designed for therapeutic uses of ionising radiation (generally B radiations) to a specific disease sites on the body.

A branch of pharmacy which deals with the manufacturing and dispensing of radioactive materials or radiopharmaceuticals is referred to radio pharmacy. Radiopharmaceuticals are used as diagnostic purpose or as therapeutic purpose. Radiopharmaceuticals that are used for therapeutic and diagnostic purpose also impact adversely the healthy cells or parts of the body.

Units of Radioactivity: Radioactivity is measured in the following units:

1. Curie
2. Roentgen (R)
3. Exposure Rate Constant
4. Roentgen Equivalent Man (REM)
5. RAD

1. Curie: The amount of radioactive substance present or the strength of its source is described in Curie (Ci). It directly depends upon the rate of radioactive decay, shown by a radionuclide. Curie may be defined as the quantity of radioactive substance which undergoes the same number of disintegrations in unit time as that of 1gm of radium which is equal to 3.7×10^{10} disintegrations per second.

Thus,

1 Curie = 3.7×10^{10} disintegrations per second (dps) or (37 trillion decays)

2. Roentgen (R): The term Roentgen (R) is described as the radiation exposure, which is the amount of air it ionises. In the International System of Units, the coulomb/kilogram (c/kg) describes radiation exposure.

$$1 R = 2.58 \times 10^{-4} \ Ckg^{-1} \ (C=Coulomb).$$

3. Exposure Rate Constant: It refers to the rate in roentgens per hour at 1m distance from 1curie. It is about one-tenth of the dose at a distance of 1 foot from 1 curie.

4. Roentgen Equivalent Man (REM): It REM refers to the unit of radiation dosage applied to human for therapeutic purpose. The dose in REM is equal to the dose in RADS multiplied by quality factor and the distribution factor.

5. Relative Biological Effectiveness (RBE): Since the effect of given radiation on biological system depends upon the type of radiation a unit known as RBE has been introduced. This expresses the relative effects of radiations α, β and γ on the biological system.

6. RAD: This term is used to describe the absorbed radiation dose. It denotes the specific amount of energy absorbed in a medium like human tissues. In the International System of Units, the Gray (Gy) describes absorbed radiation dose.

$$1 \text{ gray} = 100 \text{ RAD}$$
$$1 \text{ rad} = 10^{-2} Jkg^{-1}$$

The energy absorption equivalent of one roentgen in air has been 0.87 RAD and for water it has been 0.97 RAD.

Q.2. What is Half-life of Radioactive elements?

Half-Life: Half-life ($t_{1/2}$) is the time period in which a substance is reduced by 50% of its initial amount. Radioactive decay or nuclear decay is first order reaction and does not depend on concentration of material.

The radioactive or nuclear decay is a highly irregular phenomenon. If a radionuclide is taken and number of disintegrations is measured per second. the results obtained show that after a time period, half of the original active atoms disintegrate leaving behind the other half. Now, the number of disintegrations per second will also be the half of original value. Thus, the half-life is the time in which a radioactive substance decays to its half quantity. This time remains constant, regardless of the quantity of the substance present initially.

$$\text{Half-life } (t_{1/2}) = 0.693/\lambda$$

Where, λ is disintegration constant in unit of sec^{-1}.

Examples of radioactive isotopes and their half-life:

Radioactive Isotopes	Half-life
Polonium-212	3×10^{-7} seconds
Iodine-131	8 days
P-32	14.3 days
Uranium-238	4.5×10^{4} years
Zn-65	165 days
Na-22	2.6 years

It is the half-life of a radionuclide substance that determines its pharmaceutical importance. Successful experiments cannot be conveniently carried out due to very short half-life.

On the other hand, if half-life is long. the substance is not altered under any chemical or biological conditions, therefore, it is the most desirable property.

Q.3. What is Decay Constant?

Decay Constant: Let an element 'A' disintegrate into another element 'B'. Initially (at t=0), the element 'A' has N_0 number of atoms; as the time passes, the element 'A' disintegrates into 'B'. Thus, the number of atoms of element "A" continuously decreases. Let N be the number of atoms of 'A' which does not disintegrate in time t.

Thus, **A → B**

At, t=0 N_0

At, t=tN

If dN atoms of 'A' disintegrates in a small time dt, the rate of disintegration (i.e., rate of decrease) of 'A' prime into 'B' which is also called activity is equal to -dN/dt which is proportional to N. i.e.,

I – dN/dt α N

Or – dN/dt = λN..... (1)

Here, λ is a proportionality constant which is defined as a radioactive or decay or disintegration constant.

The disintegration rate is presented with a negative sign because as the time passes, the intensity and the number of atoms of 'A' reduces.

According to the equation (1), radioactive constant or decay or disintegration constant (2) can be given as:

$$\gamma = \frac{-\,dN \,/\, dt}{N}$$

Thus, radioactive constant is the ratio of the amount of substances which disintegrates in a unit time to the amount of the substances present.

Q.4. Define Radiation. Give properties of α (Alpha), β (Beta) and γ (Gamma) radiation with application of Radiation.

Radiation: In radiation, energy emitted by a body travels through a medium or space and is ultimately absorbed by another body.

The radioactive isotopes release charged particles of matter (i.e., α- or β- particles) as radiation; and sometimes after emission of charged particles, the nucleus is left with large energy. This amount of energy is dissolute in the form of gamma rays, which are electromagnetic type of radiation.

Properties of α, β, γ radiations: All substances are made atoms. These have electrons around the outside, and a nucleus in the middle. The nucleus consists of protons and neutrons and is extremely small. In some types of atom, the nucleus is unstable, and will decay into a more stable atom. This radioactive decay is completely spontaneous.

When an unstable nucleus decays, there are three ways that it can do so. It may give out:

1. Alpha particles(α)
2. Beta particles (β)
3. Gamma particles (γ)

Properties of Alpha Radiation: The characteristic features of alpha particles are:

1. These particles are equivalent to the nuclei of helium atoms (i.e., ^4_2He).
2. Alpha particles are positively charged and heavy.
3. They travel in air to a few centimetres and may penetrate up to 1mm of body tissues.
4. They are highly energetic particles and have energy up to 4MeV

    e.g.,$^{226}Ra \rightarrow ^{222}Ra + ^4He$
5. Alpha-emitter isotopes are not useful in pharmaceutical formulations.

Properties of Beta Radiation: The characteristic features of beta particles are:

1. Their mass is equal to an electron (approximately 1/4800 of a mass unit).
2. They are mostly negatively charged (negatron or electron), but rarely may also be positively charged (positron).
3. In air they may travel up to a few meters and may penetrate the body tissues about a centimetre.
4. The maximum energy exhibited by beta particles (E_{max}) is 1.5MeV and mean energy ($\bar{E}$) is 0.6MeV,

   e.g., $_{11}^{24}Mg \rightarrow {}_{12}^{24}Mg + \beta^-$

Properties of Gamma Radiation: The characteristic features of gamma particles are:

1. Gamma particles are similar to X-radiation.
2. These particles react with matter and behave like discrete packets (quanta) of energy, referred to as photons.
3. It is an electromagnetic radiation therefore does not have any mass or charge and travels with the speed of light.
4. Gamma particles are high energy particles, typically 2MeV.
5. These particles have high penetration power and can pass through several feet of solid matter.

Applications of Radiations: Radiations are widely used in various areas of research and development; some of them are given as:

1. Radiations are used for diagnostic purposes, for example, X-rays are used to find out any injury of bone.
2. Radiation has power to destroy tissues, thus they easily destroy bacteria and other microorganisms. This property is used for food preservation without the aid of chemicals and refrigeration.
3. Various radioactive isotopes are used to supply power to satellites and provide electricity for space laboratories.
4. They are utilised for estimating the degree of air pollution.
5. The archaeologists use radiations to determine the age and authenticity of the ancient artefacts, **e.g.,** C^{16} isotopes are used to determine the age of earth.

Q.5. Write a brief note on methods of Measurement of Radioactivity with diagram.

Measurement of Radioactivity: The radioactivity of alpha, beta and gamma particles can be measured by the help of various techniques. These techniques involve detection and counting of either protons or individual particles.

The radiation detectors are divided into two distinct categories:

1. Detectors Based on Ion Collection
   a) **Gas filled detectors**
      i)   Electroscopes,
      ii)   Ion chambers,
      iii) Proportional counters,

iv)   Geiger counters

b) Solid state detectors

i)   Barrier-state detectors,

ii)   Lithium-drifted detectors

2. Detectors Based on Photon Collection

a) Sodium iodide scintillation counters,

b) Liquid scintillation counters.

The detection and measurement of radioactive radiation can be done by many methods which are stated above, but in modern practice following equipment are used:

1. Ionisation chamber,
2. Geiger-Muller counter,
3. Scintillation counter.

1. Ionisation Chamber: Ionisation chamber simply measures the radiation strength. It is filled with two metallic plates, separated by air. On passing the radiation through the chamber, the atoms of air molecules are knocked off and the positive ions are formed. The electrons move towards the anode while positive ions towards the cathode. This results to the passage of mild current between the plates, which is measured with the help of an ammeter.

Fig. Ionisation Chamber

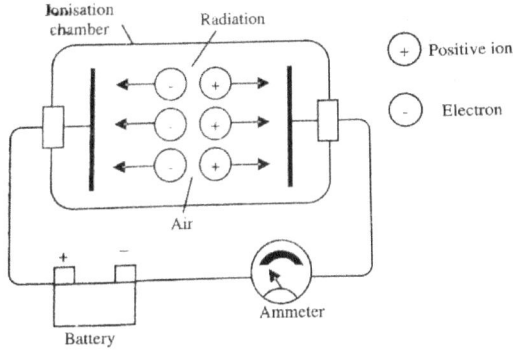

The strength of current helps in the determination of radiation passing through the ionisation chamber. The total amount of charge passing between the plates in a given time is measured by dosimeter, which is present in the ionisation chamber. This is proportional to the total amount of radiation that has gone through the chamber.

2. Geiger-Muller Counter: The rate of emission of a- or B-particles can be detected and measured by the Geiger-Muller Counter. It comprises of a cylindrical metal tube which acts as a cathode, and for anode a wire is placed centrally. The metal tube has very low pressure of around 0.1atm and is filled with argon gas.

A potential difference of 1000 volts is maintained across the electrodes. The a- or B-particle enters the tube through the mica window and the argon atoms present in tube gets ionised along the path of α- or β-particles.

The positively charged argon ions (Ar^+) move towards the cathode while the negatively charged electrons move towards the anode. The circuit is completed in very short duration of time (in microseconds), after which an electrical pulse is generated which is recorded in the automatic counter. The intensity of radioactivity can be measured by the pulse generated per minute from the radioactive material.

Fig. Geiger-Muller Counter

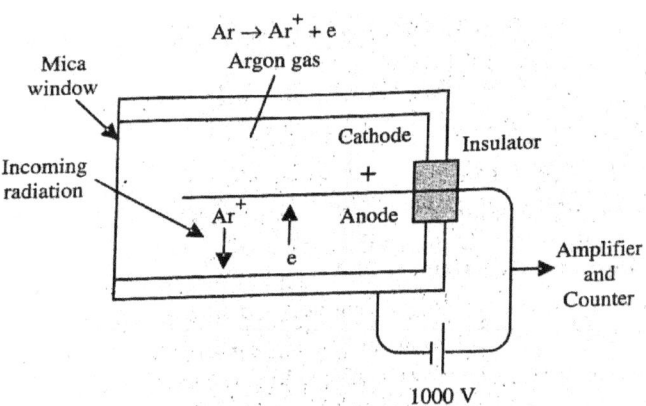

3. Scintillation Counter: As the name indicates, scintillation counter works on detecting a flash or scintillation of light, which is produced when a charged particle, or gamma ray, strikes on either fluorescent screen or on some specific type of crystals. Sodium iodide, caesium iodide, anthracene, and certain plastics are the material of choice for typical scintillators. One side of the scintillator is cemented to which the photomultiplier tube is attached and acts as photocathode. The vacuum tube consists of multiple electrodes, called dynodes. These dynodes are kept at high voltage in increasing manner.

The photocathode produces electrons (photoelectron) which are accelerated towards the first dynode. The photoelectron strikes on first dynode with large amount of kinetic energy, resulting in emission more electrons. This process is continued towards the second and third dynode and so on. and the multiplication of electrons continued.

Fig. Scintillation Counter

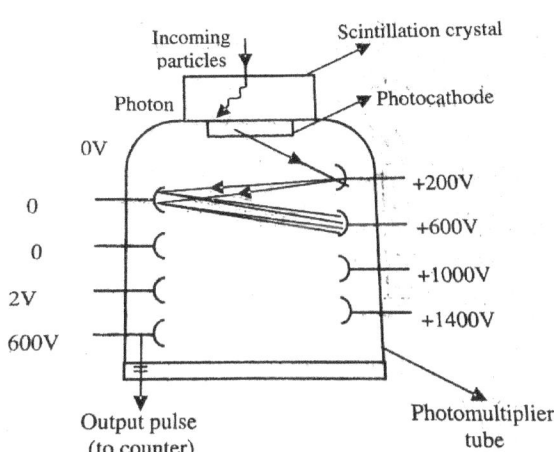

scintillator is struck by gamma rays or by charged particles, the molecules of scintillator gets excited and emits energy as light for returning When a to their ground state. This emitted light is incident on the photocathode of the photomultiplier and emits photoelectron. Since the potential difference of each dynode increases in successive manner, there occurs successive increment in electrons as they finally reach the ultimate dynode. Due to this multiplication, a weak pulse is also amplified up to 10-10 times, before reaching to the counting equipment. The output electrical pulse is proportional to the energy of the incident particle or photons.

Small amount of impurities (activators) are also added to the crystal for reducing self-absorption of light and for enhancing the photon emission probability. Thallium is the most commonly used activator.

In a Geiger-Muller counter, the crystal used as a scintillator is denser than the gas used, therefore it acts as an efficient detector. Thallium-activated sodium iodide is very efficient in detecting gamma rays. Anthracene crystal which is not very sensitive to gamma rays is used for the detection B-rays.

Q.6. What are Radioisotopes. Classify Them with Examples of some frequently used radioisotopes.

Radioisotopes: A radioisotope is an atom with an unstable nucleus. This nucleus carries large amount of energy which is utilised either by a newly-formed radiation particle within the nucleus, or by an atomic electron.

An element has different isotopes; atomic nuclei of these isotopes carry the same number of protons but the number of neutrons varies. Thus, radioisotopes are atoms with an unstable combination of neutrons and protons.

Radioisotopes also have medicinal importance, for example, the cancer cells growth may be inhibited by radiations of cobalt-60. Some radioisotopes are used as markers for diagnosing diseases, and are also used in research on metabolic processes. **For example,** hyperthyroidism is effectively treated using iodine-131; Heliobacter pylori (the bacteria causing ulcers) can be detected in a breath test using carbon-14.

Before using a radioisotope for diagnostic and therapeutic purpose, it is added in small quantity to large quantities of the stable element.

Such radioisotopes chemically behave like an ordinary isotope. Though, any detector device like Geiger counter may trace presence of even small amount of radioactive isotopes in such compounds

Classification: The following two categories of radioisotopes are available:

1. **Stable Radioisotopes:** These isotopes (e.g., C, CI", H' (protium), H (deuterium), etc.) are and do not radiations.

2. **Radioactive Radioisotopes:** These are either naturally occurring (e.g., uranium, radium, etc.) or artificially produced unstable isotopes. They emit radiation to lose energy. This phenomenon of emission of radiation is known as radioactivity and such compounds are radioactive compounds or radioactive isotopes.

Examples of Radioisotopes: Examples of some frequently used radioisotopes are:

1. **Carbon Element:** Carbon has three isotopes:

   i) **Carbon-12 ($^{12}_6C$):** It has six protons and six neutrons. It is a stable isotope with atomic number 6 and atomic mass or mass number 12.

   ii) **Carbon-13 ($^{13}_6C$):** It has six protons and seven neutrons in its nucleus. It is also a stable isotope with atomic number 6 and atomic mass 13.

   iii) **Carbon-14 ($^{14}_6C$):** It has six protons and eight neutrons in its nucleus. It is an unstable isotope with atomic number 6 and atomic mass 14. It has radioactive property and hence is a radioisotope.

The above mentioned all three isotopes of carbon has same atomic number, i.e., 6, while their atomic mass is different. They have same chemical properties.

2. **Iron Element:** These are of two types:

Types	Example
Stable	$^{54}_{26}Fe$, $^{56}_{26}Fe$, $^{57}_{26}Fe$, $^{58}_{6}Fe$
Unstable	$^{55}_{26}Fe$, $^{59}_{26}Fe$

All isotopes of iron have same atomic number, i.e., 26, but they differ in atomic mass (54, 56, 57, 58, and 59). They have same chemical properties. Iron-55(Fe) and iron-59 (Fe) are unstable radioactive isotopes.

3. **Phosphorus Element:** It has two isotopes:

i) Phosphorus-31($^{31}_{15}P$): It has 15 protons and 16 neutrons. It is a stable isotope with atomic number 15 and atomic mass 31.

ii) Phosphorus-32 ($^{32}_{15}P$): It has 15 protons and 17 neutrons. It is an unstable radioisotope with atomic number 15 and atomic mass 32.

4. **Iodine Element:** Iodine has two isotopes:

i) Iodine-127: It has 53 protons and 74 neutrons in its nucleus. It is a stable isotope atomic number 53 and atomic mass 127.

ii) Iodine-131($^{131}_{53}I$): It has 53 protons and 78 neutrons in its nucleus. It is an unstable, radioactive isotope with atomic number 53 and atomic mass 131.

Q.7. Write about I^{131} as Radioisotopes.

Sodium Iodide (I^{131}): Iodide I^{131}is a radiopharmaceutical substance used in the treatment of malignant thyroid. The ionising radiations of iodide I^{131} are absorbed by the thyroid tissue. Tissue damage results due to direct exposure because the molecules dissociate due to the ionisation and excitation. The sodium iodide I^{131} emits about 90% of β-radiation and the remaining 10% is the γ-radiation.

Mechanism of Action: The iodide enters in the thyroid through the sodium/iodide symporter and accumulates there. Here it oxidises into iodine and emits radiations. These β-radiations emitted by sodium iodideI^{131} destroy the thyroid tissue.

Properties: Sodium iodide is a colourless solution having a pH between 7-10. Half-life of sodium iodideI^{131} is 8.4 days. It emits β- and γ-radiations. About 99% of its energy released in the form of radiations is expanded within 56 days.

Assay: Using an appropriate counting instrument sodium iodideI^{131}is assayed by comparing its activity with a standardI^{131}solution. It is also tested for the purity radionuclide and radiochemical.

Uses:

1. Hyperthyroidism and some cases of thyroid malignancy are treated using sodium iodide I^{131} Sodium iodide mainly acts on thyroid gland.

2. In cases of hyperthyroidism (thyroid gland becomes hyperactive), the radioactive iodine emits radiation which destroys some cells of thyroid gland and normalises its activity.

3. After the surgical removal of cancerous thyroid gland, radio iodide is given in large doses to destroy the remaining diseased thyroid tissue and the diseased neighbouring tissues.

4. In small doses radio iodide is used for diagnosis.

5. It is used to detect normal functioning of thyroid gland and detecting tumour.

Toxicity: Sialadenitis, chest pain, tachycardia, iododerma, itching, skin rashes, hives, hypothyroidism, hyperthyroidism, thyrotoxic crisis, hypoparathyroidism, and local swelling are some adverse effects of sodium iodideI^{131}occurring during the treatment of Benign disease.

Radiation sickness, bone marrow depression, anaemia, leucopoenia, thrombocytopenia, blood dyscrasia, leukaemia, solid cancers, lacrimal gland dysfunction, salivary gland dysfunction, congenital hypothyroidism, chromosomal abnormalities, cerebral oedema, radiation pneumonitis, and pulmonary fibrosis are some severe dose related adverse effects which sodium iodide I^{131}produces while treating malignancy.

Q.8. Write a note on Production of Isotopes.

Production of Isotopes: the radionuclides used in nuclear medicine are produced artificially by the following methods.

1. Cyclotrons
2. Nuclear Reactors
3. Radionuclide Generators

1.Cyclotrons:

i) Radionuclides are produced from cyclotrons when high-energy charged particles are bombarded on the stable nuclei.

ii) The resultant radionuclides are neutron deficit, and therefore decompose by positron emission or electron capture.

iii) For therapeutic and diagnostic purpose specialised hospital-based cyclotrons have been developed to produce positron-emitting radionuclides for Positron Emission Tomography Cyclotrons are positioned near the PET imager due to their short half-lives. (PET).

2. Nuclear Reactors:

i) Radionuclides of clinical significance are produced by some specialised nuclear reactors from fission products or by activating neutrons of a stable material.

ii) The fission products of U235 and other stable isotopes (carrier) are separated from each other by chemical means. These stable isotopes function as carrier and are radionuclide.

3. Radionuclide Generators:

i) A radionuclide generator system holds the parent in a way that releases less intense products which can be used for clinical purpose.

ii) The radionuclide which has been frequently used in nuclear medicine is technetium-99m.

iii) Due to their short half-life (6 hours), it is impractical to store them.

iv) However, this supply problem can be resolved by using parent Mo-99 with a longer half-life (67 hours) and continually producing Tc-99m.

Q.9. Give Diagnostic and Analytical Applications of Radioisotopes.

Diagnostic and Analytical Applications of Radioisotopes: The radioisotopes are widely used in the field of diagnosis and analysis:

1. **Diagnostic Applications:** The radioisotopes are used for diagnosing of various organs, **e.g.,** heart, liver, kidney, etc.
   Some of the major diagnostic applications are discussed in table

Organ or Tissue	Radionuclide and their complexes used for Diagnosis
Heart	Thallium T1-201 chloride injection is used for myocardial imaging and for early detection of infarction. The ^{99m}Tc-tetracycline and ^{99m}Tc-pyrophosphate are used for infarct scanning

Thyroid	Iodine[131] (sodium iodide) is used for thyroid scanning
Liver	Iodine[131] is used for hepatobiliary imaging. ^{99m}Tc-HIDA, ^{99m}Tc-mebrofen, ^{99m}Tc-sulphur colloid and ^{113m}Tc are other agents used for diagnosis of liver diseases
Kidney	^{99m}TC-ascorbate and ^{99m}TC dimercaptosuccinate are useful for kidney imaging. Sodium iodohippurate with is used for demonstration of renal insufficiency
Tumours	Galium-67 citrate is used for evaluating patients with Hodgkin's disease, melanoma, lung carcinoma and Burkett's lymphoma
Brain	^{99m}Tc-pertechnetate is used for brain imaging
Lungs	Iodinated I[131] serum albumin is used to see the pulmonary vasculature through perfusion lung scanning

2. **Analytical Applications:** Some of the major analytical applications of radioisotopes are:

a) **Analytical Procedures:** Some new techniques of analysis and separation using radioisotopes are being developed due to their speed and sensitivity. **For example,** determination of efficiency of complexing agents used in chromatography

b) **Radio-Isotope Dilution Analysis:** A compound of desired purity can be isolated using complex samples but it cannot be easily recovered quantitatively. This problem can be resolved by using radioisotope dilution analysis.

In this method, a trace compound (Mt) of known amount and activity (c) is added to a sample (Ms) with an unknown mass (M) of the desired component. After equilibrium is attained, the desired compound in its purest form is separated and its activity (C) and mass (m) are determined. Mass of the desired substance in the sample is given as:

$$M = m.C/c - Mt$$

c) **Recovery Indication in Analysis:** The process involved in recovery indication is same as the distribution analysis. The only difference is that in recovery indication the radioactive labelled material added at the outset is almost of negligible mass. This minimises the losses due to volatilisation and adsorption.

d) **Radioimmunoassay:** A large number of compounds can be assayed by radioimmunoassay, i.e., digoxin, insulin, etc.

e) **Solubility Determination:** The solubility of a radioactive labelled substance (with low solubility) can be determined by preparing its saturated solution. An aliquot of this solution is taken and its activity is compared with that of the standard labelled material.

f) Activation Analysis: Presence of low concentration of some elements in a sample (**e.g, tissues**) can be detected and measured analytically by subjecting the sample to neutrons. The sample along with the standard is placed in a nuclear reactor, so that both get irradiated in a similar fashion.

$$\frac{\text{Activity in sample}}{\text{Activity in standard}} = \frac{\text{Mass of element in sample}}{\text{Mass of standard}}$$

Since the activities of sample and standard are measured, the mass of standard is known, so that the mass of the sample can be calculated.

g) **Enzyme Assays:** Highly specific, sensitive, and accurate enzymes are assayed using radiochemical methods.

h) **Receptors Assays:** The tissues and organs of human body comprise of various receptor systems which can be assayed by using radioisotopes. For example, assay of oestrogen receptor site in breast cancer aids in hormonal treatment of breast cancer.

Q.10. What are Radiopharmaceuticals. Give ideal diagnostic properties with Storage condition of radiopharmaceuticals.

Radiopharmaceuticals: Radiopharmaceuticals are specially designed products that are used therapeutically for treatment and diagnosis. Their usages are very restricted and are primarily used for diagnostic purpose.

The radiopharmaceuticals get distributed in the body and emit radiations. These radiations are photographed to detect internal injury, abnormal cell growth, etc. The radiation exposure is kept very low.

In X-ray, low intensity electromagnetic rays (gamma rays) are used that penetrate the body tissue but cannot penetrate bones; thus, forming pictures of bones. By analysing these X-ray images, any injury, fracture or abnormal growth of bones can be detected.

In the field of nuclear medicine, radiopharmaceuticals are used as tracers for diagnosis and for treating various diseases. Many radiopharmaceuticals use Technetium (Tc-99m). Thirty-one different radiopharmaceuticals based on Tc- 99m are listed for imaging and functional studies of the brain, myocardium, thyroid, lungs, liver, gallbladder, kidneys, skeleton, blood, and tumours.

Ideal Diagnostic Radiopharmaceutical: A radiopharmaceutical should have the following properties in order to be used for diagnostic purpose:

1. **Types of Emission:** Only gamma particles should be emitted by a since a- and $\square$-particles remain undetected and deliver a very high radiation dose.
2. **Energy of Gamma Rays:**
   i) Ideal: 100-250keV, **e.g.,**^{99m}Tc, ^{123}I, ^{111}In
   ii) Suboptimal:$<100keV$, **e.g.,**^{201}TI
   $>250keV$, **e.g.,**^{67}Ga and ^{131}I

3. **Photon Abundance:** It should be high to minimise imaging time.

4. **Target to Non-Target Ratio:** It should be high to maximise efficacy of diagnosis and minimise the radiation dose to patients.

5. **Easy Availability:** It should be readily available and inexpensive, **e.g.,** ^{11}C and ^{99m}Tc.

6. **Patient Safety:** It should exhibit no toxicity to the patient.

7. **Preparation and Quality Control:**

   i) Should be simple with little manipulation,

   ii) No complicated equipment required, and

   iii) No time-consuming steps.

Storage Conditions: The radiopharmaceuticals are stored in airtight containers in a shielded place. This place should be organised as per the national and international regulations set forth for the storage of radioactive substances. Personnel should not be exposed to any primary or secondary emissions.

The containers of radiopharmaceuticals may become dark due to irradiation, although this does not indicate that the substance has degraded. Radioactive substances are suggested to be used within a short time period and the expiry period should also be clearly mentioned. The parenteral radiopharmaceuticals should not lose their purity during storage; thus, optimum storage conditions should be maintained.

Q.11. Write a short note on Hazards and Precautions in handling of radiopharmaceuticals.

Hazards of Radiopharmaceuticals: The radioactive particles affect the biological tissues; these depend on various factors like:

1. The ability of the radiation to penetrate tissues,
2. The energy of radiation,
3. Type of particular tissue,
4. Surface area exposed, and
5. Dose rate of the radiation.

The destructive aspect of radioactivity is directly related to its interaction with molecules present in the tissue to form abnormal amounts of ions and/or free radicals:

1. The chemical entities can lead to initiation of free chain reactions or changes in the local pH, which may liberate peroxides or other toxic compounds.
2. Such events may lead to unfavourable environment for the tissues, which may cause necrosis and finally destruction of body tissues.
3. Tissues present in human body are made up of about 70% water, which acts as the most reactive species for the ionising radiation, apart from the other biochemicals involved in the reaction. An illustration of free radical formation and reaction to form hydrogen peroxide is shown in the given reaction.

4. Free radicals produced by water may lead to the abstraction of radicals from other compounds, yielding various potentially toxic substances that can cause alteration in DNA sequencing.

In low doses (below 1 radiation), the radiopharmaceuticals may alter individual cells (damaged either singly in small numbers), induce cancer cells, and adversely affect embryonic development.

The following hazards of radiation exposure and the relative risk of such effects are observed:

1. Induction of Cancer: Induction of cancer is the biggest threat for those who are exposed to even low-level radiations. Radiation induces oncogene which remains in dormant state. Activation of oncogene causes various types of cancers like breast cancer, thyroid cancer, lung cancer, leukaemia, alimentary tract cancer, etc.

2. Genetic Effects: Genetic risks in humans are largely based on the studies performed on animals, since there is no significant demonstration of radiation induced gene mutation in humans. Thus, the risk of a genetic defect in the child of a patient who had undergone a diagnostic test using radionuclides is insignificant.

3. Effect on the Embryo: Since, the developing embryo is sensitive to radiations, during the diagnostic procedures the exposure rate for the embryo is kept under 5rads. At this rate the risk is negligible. While at the exposure rate of above 15rads, risk of malformation increases significantly. At higher

doses embryo may experience death, malformation, and retarded growth. The significance of these effects increases with the increase in dose. The gestation stage of the mother during the irradiation is very important for the determination of the effects, as the organ system is highly sensitive at the time of organogenesis.

4. Lactation: During lactation there is high risk of using radiopharmaceutical, as it may reach to child via milk. To overcome this problem a safe interval of time is taken between administration of radiopharmaceutical and breast feeding, **e.g.,** when Tc-99m is administered, breast feeding should be discontinued for 24 hours.

Precautions in Handling of Radiopharmaceuticals: Great care has to be taken in handling and storage of radioactive material for protecting people and personnel handling it. The precautions that should be taken are:

1. The radioactive material should not contaminate the working area.

2. In case the radioactive material is liquid, the material should be carried in trays having absorbent tissue paper for absorbing any accidental spillage.

3. While handling liquid radioactive materials, rubber gloves should be used.

4. Mouth operated pipettes should not be used. Moreover, it should be ensured that the glass apparatus should be

inactivated, before their usage. Before disposition of radioactive material, they should have very low activity; otherwise they are stored till the activity reduces to safer levels.

5. Activities such as smoking, eating, and drinking are strictly prohibited in the area of radioactive work.

6. Forceps should be used while handling the radioactive emitter.

7. Shielding devices should be used sufficiently.

8. The radioactive material should be stored in well-labelled containers using bricks (for shielding). It is preferred to store radioactive material in a remote corner.

9. The area in which the radioactive material is stored should be monitored constantly.

10. The disposal of radioactive material is done with utmost care.

Q.12. Give in detail note on application of radiopharmaceuticals.

Pharmaceutical Applications of Radioactive Substances: For medical purpose, radiopharmaceuticals can be used by the following two different ways:

1. **Therapeutic Applications**
2. **Diagnostic Applications**

1. **Therapeutic Applications:** The therapeutic effect of radiopharmaceuticals utilises the destructive features of the radiations. These radiations destroy abnormally multiplied cells and further inhibit the formation of new cells and tissues. Hence, it is frequently

used in the treatment of disorders like cancers which involves extensive cellular malfunction.

Isotopes can be selected on the basis of the following factors:

i. Characteristics of the radiation required for treatment,
ii. Types of radiation,
iii. Energy and intensity of radiation, and
iv. Types of tissues

Both external and internal radiation sources are utilised in the therapy:

i. External Sources

a) Teletherapy Sources:^{60}Co, ^{137}Cs and neutral charged particles.
b) Surface Sources:^{90}Sr. ^{32}P (beta emitters)
c) Extracorporeal Irradiation:^{60}Co, ^{90}Sr. ^{90}Y.

ii. Internal Sources

a) Infusion:^{196}Au, ^{32}p
b) Interstitial Implant:^{192}Ir, ^{125}I
c) Selectively Absorbed or Concentrated:^{32}p, ^{131}I, ^{90}Y

The therapeutic preparations containing radioisotopes are collectively referred to as radiopharmaceuticals,

for example:

1. **Teletherapy:** This technique mostly utilises highly active gamma- emitting isotopes (as high as 2000°C) like ^{60}Co or^{137}Cs. these isotopes are used to treat lesions by applying them directly on the affected area.

2. **Implantation Therapy:** In this technique sealed radioactive sources are introduced directly into the tumour tissues.

Isotopes like ^{60}Co, ^{192}Ir, ^{198}Au, and ^{182}Ta are typically used in this way.

3. **Surface or Contact Therapy:** Pure beta emitters like ^{32}P and ^{90}Sr are used for treating dermatological and ophthalmological tumour, whereas bladder tumours are treated by introducing ^{32}P isotope in the affected area.

4. **Extracorporeal Irradiation:**^{60}Co sources are used to determine the depletion of lymphocytes in blood. This depletion may alter the immunological response. **Other examples** of different radioisotopes used in the treatment:

   i. **Iridium (^{192}Ir):** It emits beta and gamma radiations and produces local destructive effects on cells.

   ii. **Sodium Phosphate (^{32}P):** It is used in the treatment of polycythaemia and decreases the rate of erythrocyte formation. It is also used in the treatment of chronic granulocytic leukaemia.

   iii. **Yttrium (^{90}Y):** It has a $t_{1/2}$ of 64 hours. It emits only a single beta particle (2.27 MeV) with no gamma radiation. It can chelate with N-hydroxy ethylenediamine tetra acetic acid and thus can be localised in the bone. This chelate has been used to treat leukaemia and multiple myeloma.

   iv. **Iodine (^{125}I):** It has a t2 of 60 days and is used for permanent implant and treatment of deep-seated tumours like tumour of chest which cannot be removed by surgery.

3. Diagnostic Applications: The diagnostic applications of radiopharmaceuticals are summarised in the table.

Diagnostic Purpose	Radio Pharmaceuticals
1. Brain Imaging i. Evaluate cerebral function ii. Evaluate cerebral perfusion	To-99m labelled lipophilic agents Ceretec, Neurolite
2. Thyroid Imaging i. Determine function (as % uptake of iodine) ii. Evaluate shape, size and location of thyroid gland	I-131 sodium

3. Heart Imaging
 	
i. Assess myocardial perfusion
ii. Determine myocardial function
   a) Wall motion
   b) Ejection fraction
	TI-201 chloride

4. Gastric Imaging i. Gastric Imaging/ Reflux/ Aspiration ii. GI Bleeding iii. Hepatobiliary Imaging iv. Liver/Spleen	Tc-99m SC Tc-99m SC, Tc-99m RBC Tc-99m IDA compounds Tc-99m SC
5. Bone Imaging i. Assess trauma, bone pain, primary bone tumour, infection &prosthetics ii. Detect and stage metastatic disease	Tc-99m phosphate compounds
6. Pulmonary Imaging i. Evaluation of pulmonary ventilation	Te-99m DTPA, Xe-133 gas Tc-99m labelled MAA

ii. Evaluation of pulmonary perfusion	
7. Renal Imaging i. Assessment of flow and function ii. Evaluation of renal morphology	Tc-99m labelled agents for filtration and secretion Te-99m labelled morphology agents
8. Infection Imaging Localise internal sources of infection	Tc-99m or In-111 labelled white blood cells Ga-67
9. Tumour Imaging i. Evaluating location and spreading of tumor ii. Evaluating metabolic activity of tumour cells	Ga-67 F-18 FdG
10. Bone Pain Palliation Palliative treatment for pain associated with metastatic disease to the bone	Sr-89, Sm-153

Bibliography

1. Block J.H., Roche E., Sonie T., Wilson C., Inorganic, Medicinal and Pharmaceutical Chemistry, Lea and Febiger.

2. Atherden L. M., Bentley's and Driver's Text Book of Pharmaceutical Chemistry, Oxford University Press.

3. Pharmacopoeia of India.

4. Miessler G. L., Tarr D. A., Inorganic Chemistry, Dorling Kinderley (India) Pvt. Ltd. (Pearson Education).

5. Das Ishwar, Sharma Archana, Agarwal R. Namita, An Introduction to Physical Chemistry, New Age International.

6. Remington: The Science and Practice of Pharmacy Pharmaceutical Sciences Vol. I and III, Mark Publishing Company, U.S.A.

7. Vogel A.I., Text Book of Quantitative Inorganic Analysis, Person Education.

8. http://www.scribd.com

9. http://nsdl.niscair.res.in

10. http://www.pharmainfo.net

11. http://www.slidshare.net

12. http://www.pharmpress.com

13. http://www.authorstream.com

14. http://www.usp.org

15. http://www.ipc.gov.in